BACTEREMIA

Publication Number 899
AMERICAN LECTURE SERIES

A Monograph in

The BANNERSTONE DIVISION *of*
AMERICAN LECTURES IN CLINICAL MICROBIOLOGY

Edited by

ALBERT BALOWS, Ph.D.
Chief, Bacteriology Branch
Laboratory Division
Center for Disease Control
Atlanta, Georgia

BACTEREMIA

LABORATORY AND
CLINICAL ASPECTS

Edited by

ALEX C. SONNENWIRTH, Ph.D.
Division of Microbiology
The Jewish Hospital of St. Louis
Departments of Microbiology and Pathology
Washington University School of Medicine, St. Louis, Missouri

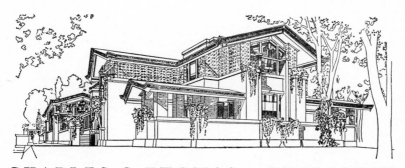

CHARLES C THOMAS · PUBLISHER
Springfield · Illinois · U.S.A.

Published and Distributed Throughout the World by
CHARLES C THOMAS • PUBLISHER
BANNERSTONE HOUSE
301-327 East Lawrence Avenue, Springfield, Illinois, U.S.A.

© 1973, by CHARLES C THOMAS • PUBLISHER
ISBN 0-398-02829X
Library of Congress Catalog Card Number: 73-207

With THOMAS BOOKS *careful attention is given to all details of
manufacturing and design. It is the Publisher's desire to present books
that are satisfactory as to their physical qualities and artistic possibilities
and appropriate for their particular use.* THOMAS BOOKS *will be true
to those laws of quality that assure a good name and good will.*

Printed in the United States of America
W-1

CONTRIBUTORS

Raymond C. Bartlett, M.D.
Division of Microbiology
Department of Pathology
Hartford Hospital
Hartford, Connecticut

Sydney M. Finegold, M.D.
Veterans Administration
Wadsworth General Hospital
Los Angeles, California

Donald A. Goldmann, M.D.
Department of Health, Education, and Welfare
Health Services and Mental Health Administration
Center for Disease Control
Epidemiology Program
Bacterial Diseases Branch
Hospital Infections Section
Atlanta, Georgia

and

Division of Infectious Disease
University of Virginia School of Medicine
Charlottesville, Virginia

Dennis G. Maki, M.D.
Department of Health, Education, and Welfare
Health Services and Mental Health Administration
Center for Disease Control
Epidemiology Program
Bacterial Diseases Branch
Hospital Infections Section
Atlanta, Georgia

and

Division of Infectious Disease
University of Virginia School of Medicine
Charlottesville, Virginia

v

Gerald L. Mandell, M.D.
Department of Health, Education, and Welfare
Health Services and Mental Health Administration
Center for Disease Control
Epidemiology Program
Bacterial Diseases Branch
Hospital Infections Section
Atlanta, Georgia

and

Division of Infectious Disease
University of Virginia School of Medicine
Charlottesville, Virginia

Frank S. Rhame, M.D.
Department of Health, Education, and Welfare
Health Services and Mental Health Administration
Center for Disease Control
Epidemiology Program
Bacterial Diseases Branch
Hospital Infections Section
Atlanta, Georgia

and

Division of Infectious Disease
University of Virginia School of Medicine
Charlottesville, Virginia

Richard Rosner, M.S.
Department of Microbiology
St. Joseph's Hospital
Paterson, New Jersey

Alex C. Sonnenwirth, Ph.D.
Division of Microbiology
The Jewish Hospital of St. Louis
Departments of Microbiology and Pathology
Washington University School of Medicine
St. Louis, Missouri

John A. Washington II, M.D.
Section of Clinical Microbiology
Mayo Clinic and Mayo Foundation
Rochester, Minnesota

FOREWORD

T HE GENESIS OF THIS SERIES, *The American Lecture Series in Clinical Microbiology,* stems from the concerted efforts of the Editor and the Publisher to provide a forum from which well-qualified and distinguished authors may present, either as a book or monograph, their views on any aspect of clinical microbiology. Our definition of clinical microbiology is conceived to encompass the broadest aspects of medical microbiology not only as it is applied to the clinical laboratory but equally to the research laboratory and to theoretical considerations. In the clinical microbiology laboratory we are concerned with differences in morphology, biochemical behavior and antigenic patterns as a means of microbial identification. In the research laboratory or when we employ microorganisms as a model in theoretical biology, our interest is often focused not so much on the above differences but rather on the similarities between microorganisms. However, it must be appreciated that even though there are many similarities between cells, there are important differences between major types of cells which set very definite limits on the cellular behavior. Unless this is understood it is impossible to discern common denominators.

We are also concerned with the relationships between microorganism and disease—any microorganism and any disease. Implicit in these relations is the role of the host which forms the third arm of the triangle microorganism, disease and host. In this series we plan to explore each of these; singly where possible for factual information and in combination for an understanding of the myriad of interrelationships that exist. This necessitates the application of basic principles of biology and may, at times, require the emergence of new theoretical concepts which will create new principles or modify existing ones. Above all, our aim is to present well-documented books which will be informative, instructive and useful, creating a sense of satisfaction to both the reader and the author.

Closely intertwined with the above _raison d'être_ is our desire to produce a series which will be read not only for the pleasure of knowledge but which will also enhance the reader's professional skill and extend his technical ability. _The American Lecture Series in Clinical Microbiology_ is dedicated to biologists— be they physicians, scientists or teachers—in the hope that this series will foster better appreciation of mutual problems and help close the gap between theoretical and applied microbiology.

This monograph, _Bacteremia: Laboratory and Clinical Aspects,_ brings into sharp focus one of today's most important areas of concern in medicine and infectious diseases. While exact figures on the prevalence and incidence of bacteremia in hospitalized patients are not available, it is universally accepted that bacteremia is one of our major medical problems. The importance of the problem is further highlighted when one recognizes that the mortality rate of patients with bacteremia runs from 20 percent to 80 percent depending to some extent on the presence or absence of shock.

In this monograph, a group of clinicians and laboratory scientists has considered several important facets of the bacteremia problem. The extent of the problem is defined by Dr. Alex Sonnenwirth; blood culture techniques, and the attending difficulties are brought to light by Dr. Raymond Bartlett. Dr. Sydney Finegold draws from his long experience and describes how the early detection of bacteremia is best approached and solved by first considering the clinical and bacteriological problems in obtaining, processing and culturing a blood specimen. Dr. John Washington presents some very startling data and describes the experience of the Mayo Clinic as it relates to anaerobic, or unusual or the more fastidious bacteria as a cause of sepsis. Richard Rosner presents his solution to blood culturing techniques which was obtained after a problem-oriented evaluation and solution in the clinical microbiology laboratory of a large, busy hospital. The final chapter by Drs. Maki, Rahme, Goldmann, and Mandell, demonstrates how the solution to one problem— improved infusion therapy—may set the stage for the emergence of another problem. The association of bacteremia with infused solutions has always been recognized but more recently it has gained worldwide prominence with several outbreaks of bacteriemia associated with the infusion of intravenous solutions reported in several countries. This monograph will enable microbiologists, physicians, epidemiologists and other health care personnel to develop a better appreciation of how the team approach to an old problem will lessen the risk and, hopefully, provide better patient care.

ALBERT BALOWS, Ph.D.
Editor, American Lecture Series
in Clinical Microbiology

PREFACE

THIS MONOGRAPH AROSE out of the Seminar on Bacteremia—
Laboratory and Clinical Aspects, held at the 1971 Annual Meeting of the American Society for Microbiology in Minneapolis, Minn. Following the seminar, the participants were made aware of a feeling among microbiologists, pathologists, internists and surgeons that a useful purpose would be served by making available the information presented and publishing it in the form of a concise reference work on various facets of bacteremia.

The individual contributions, authored by experts in the particular area about which they are writing, were considerably enlarged and brought up-to-date; references were also provided for further reading. As a result, the monograph contains a good deal of new material and new ways of looking at known data that should prove useful to those interested in microbial diseases and in better patient care.

ALEX C. SONNENWIRTH, Ph.D.

CONTENTS

BACTEREMIA

CHAPTER 1

BACTEREMIA—EXTENT OF THE PROBLEM

Alex C. Sonnenwirth

THE INCREASED INCIDENCE of bacteremia in hospital patients
that has occurred since 1935, a period during which a large
number of effective antibiotics and chemotherapeutic agents
were introduced and used intensively both for the therapy of
infectious diseases and for prophylaxis, has been extensively
documented (1, 2, 3). A changing etiologic pattern, namely a
striking rise in bacteremia due to enterobacteriaceae and other
gram-negative bacilli, with a corresponding fall in streptococcal
and pneumococcal bacteremia, has also become evident in the
last two decades (1, 2, 3, 4, 5).

The upsurge in gram-negative bacteremia has assumed truly
spectacular proportions in the last decade. Altemeier et al. (6)
reported a rise from 0.7 cases per 1,000 admissions in 1959 to
2.5 in 1965 at the University of Cincinnati Medical Center, Fried
and Vosti (7) at the Palo Alto Stanford Hospital noted an increase
from 0.7 in 1960 to 4 in 1966, while DuPont and Spink (8) at
the University of Minnesota Medical Center described a rise
from 4.9 in 1958 to 8.1 per 1,000 in 1966. The suggestion has
been made both in the United States (3, 8) and in England (9)
that a partial explanation of the increase could be the fact that
blood cultures are obtained from hospitalized patients more frequently than in previous years. Nevertheless, there is virtually
general agreement about the steady rise in the frequency of
bacteremia in American hospitals (10) as well as in Australia
(11) and England (12).

The frequency of all bacteremias in American hospitals in
1968 was conservatively estimated by Martin (10) to have been
in the range of 10 cases per 1,000 admissions and that of gram-

3

negative bacteremias, about 6 per 1,000. If such a national pro-
jection is anywhere near the mark, then there were at least one
quarter million bacteremias in 1968 in the United States with a
minimum of some 50,000 deaths. Therefore, according to Martin
(10), the published data indicate not just a number of local
institutional problems but the existence of a full-blown national
bacteremia epidemic which requires the establishment of a
national bacteremia registry, i.e. a centralized program for the
systematic collection and analysis of data concerning bacteremias
in the United States. The U.S. Center for Disease Control was
suggested as the logical organization for such an undertaking.
While no such formal operation has yet been created, the begin-
nings of a surveillance mechanism for bacteremias due to contaminated infusion fluids have been laid by the Center for
Disease Control (see Chapter 6).

Predisposing Factors and Sources of Bacteremia

The major factor responsible for the increased incidence and
changing ecology of serious bacterial infections, including bacteremia, seen at the Boston City Hospital in the period of 1935
to 1965 was presumed by Finland (3) to be the selective pressure
of the antibiotics so intensively and widely used both in therapy
and for prophylaxis. The general validity of this presumption is
underlined by the widely noted findings that bacteremias due
to organisms that continue to be susceptible to most antibiotics
and antimicrobial agents, i.e. pneumococci and group A streptococci, have declined in frequency. At the same time, bacteremias due to organisms which developed varying degrees of
resistance to a number of antibiotics or were resistant initially,
occur more frequently and with greater fatality rates (i.e.
Staphylococcus aureus, various Enterobacteriaceae, enterococci,
pseudomonads).

The emergence of antibiotic-resistant strains occurring after
the introduction and intensive use of a particular antibiotic has
been documented, among others, by Lepper *et al.* (13) in connec-
tion with erythromycin and *S. aureus*, and Finland *et al.* (1) for
chloramphenicol, kanamycin, tetracycline and *Klebsiella*.

In the studies cited, as well as in others, it was found that the highest proportions of strains resistant to the commonly used antibiotics were isolated from patients after they had antibiotic therapy. Moreover, hands and throats of patients receiving antibiotics during hospitalization were shown to be colonized with usually multiple-resistant gram-negative bacilli at high rates whereas those patients not receiving antibiotics showed practically no changes in colonization rates (14).

Numerous other factors are also involved in the rise in frequency and changing etiology of bacteremias, especially those due to gram-negative bacilli. McHenry *et al.* (15) listed them as follows: (a) aging of the population with consequent lowered ability to resist infection; (b) the widespread use of ambitious surgical and instrumental procedures; (c) prolongation of life in seriously ill patients who are particularly infection-prone, and (d) treatment (radiation, steroid or antimetabolic therapy).

Among the non-infectious diseases, liver disease (8), diabetes mellitus, malignant lymphoma, leukemias, aplastic anemia (2), and malignant neoplasms are generally recognized as predisposing especially to gram-negative bacteremia. Patients with granulocytopenia and agranulocytosis, induced either by chemotherapeutic agents or radiation therapy, are highly susceptible.

Hospital-associated cases clearly represent the major part of bacteremia cases, especially those due to gram-negative bacilli. In a series of 136 bacteremic patients, Myerowitz *et al.* (16) were able to divide these into two groups, the first representing patients who acquired bacteremia outside the hospital, and the second, a majority of the patients, composed of those who had bacteremia during hospitalization or shortly thereafter.

Various forms of (hospital-based) therapy and operative procedures are important precipitating factors of bacteremia (17). Surgical instrumentation of the genitourinary tract is probably the factor most frequently followed by gram-negative bacteremia, followed by gastrointestinal tract surgery (2, 8, 17). In such cases, the etiologic organisms often may be part of the patient's own indigenous biota, or they may represent contamination from without. Organ transplantations, radical surgical procedures and implantation of various prosthetic devices also decrease host-defense mechanisms and thus predispose to bacteremia.

Common-source outbreaks of gram-negative bacteremia in hospitals occur when fluids or equipment are contaminated by a given organism which is transferred thus to a number of patients (18). Often such organisms are of the *free-living* category (i.e. enterobacters, serratiae, pseudomonads and flavobacteria). The list of fluids, instruments and apparatus involved in common outbreaks is constantly growing: for a detailed bibliography and review, see Bassett (19). Contaminated respiratory apparatus (nebulizers, ventilators, tracheal catheters, suction apparatus), intravascular instruments (cardiac catheters and adaptors, oxygenator or heart-lung machine, plastic parts of hemodyalizer), newborns' incubators, and various fluids (hand and skin lotions, saline, eye irrigation fluids, intravenous infusion fluids) seem to be the most significant sources of such outbreaks.

The infected patient in a particular setting, e.g. surgery department, presents another important focus of infective source to other usually highly susceptible patients in the same location. Contact infection with *Klebsiella, Proteus, Pseudomonas* and other enteric organisms plays a major role in nosocomial infections and contributes to the high rate of bacteremia.

Incidence and Etiologic Agents

The experience with bacteremia in the years 1960 and 1970 at The Jewish Hospital of St. Louis, a general, university-affiliated, 530-bed hospital, was reviewed and is illustrated in Table 1-I. Despite the lack of uniformity in laboratory techniques and media employed, making comparisons difficult, the data shown indicate close similarity and agreement with rates of incidence of bacteremia and the relative frequency of etiologic agents reported by a number of investigators (3, 5, 8, 17, 20).

As shown in Table 1-I, the *total* number of blood cultures drawn at The Jewish Hospital rose from 1,238 in 1960 to 3,094 in 1970, an increase of 149 percent, whereas the admission rate increased only about 10 percent. Thus, the number of blood cultures drawn increased from 88.34/1,000 admissions in 1960 to 199.84/1,000 in 1970. Evidently, more blood cultures were

TABLE-1-I

BACTEREMIA—THE JEWISH HOSPITAL OF ST. LOUIS

Tabulation and frequency of bacteremias and of microorganisms
isolated from blood cultures*

Year	1960		1970	
Patients admitted	14,013		15,482	
Total No. blood cultures	1,238		3,094	
Positive blood cultures	120 (9.69%)		303 (9.79%)	
Bacteremic patients	79		151	
Bacteremia/1,000 admissions	5.63		9.75	

Organisms	No.	% of Orgs. Isolated	No.	% of Orgs. Isolated
Monoinfections:				
E. coli	20	25.3	37	24.5
Klebsiella	5	6.3	18	11.9
Enterobacter	4	5.0	6	3.9
Providence	1	1.2	—	—
P. mirabilis	4	5.0	5	3.3
P. morganii	—	—	3	1.9
Pseudomonas	1	1.2	11	7.3
Serratia	—	—	2	1.3
Citrobacter	1	1.2	2	1.3
Aeromonas	1	1.2	1	0.6
Acinetobacter (Mima-Herellea)	1	1.2	2	1.3
Salmonella	—	—	1	0.6
Bacteroidaceae	1	1.2	10	6.6
Total	39	49.3	98	64.5
Gram-negative bacteremia/1,000 adm.	2.71		6.33	
S. aureus	10	12.6	10	6.6
S. pneumoniae	6	7.6	4	2.6
Streptococcus viridans	12	15.1	7	4.6
Streptococcus, pyogenic	1	1.2	7	4.6
Streptococcus, Group D	2	2.5	5	3.3
Streptococcus, anaerobic	—	—	1	0.7
Listeria	1	1.2	—	—
Clostridium	2	2.5	4	2.6
Total	34	42.7	38	25.1
Gram-positive bacteremia/1,000 adm.	2.42		2.45	
Candida	2	2.5	3	1.9
N. meningitidis	1	1.2	1	0.6
Polymicrobial infections:				
G. neg. + G. neg.	—		5	
G. neg. + G. pos.	1		3	
2 G. neg. + 1 G. pos.	—		2	
3 G. neg.	2		1	
Total	3	3.8	11	7.3
Polymicrobial bacteremia/1,000 adm.	0.21		0.71	
Totals	79	100	151	100

* Cultures positive only for Staphylococcus albus, "diphtheroids" and other
organisms considered as "contaminants" are omitted.

drawn each year on a larger percentage of patients, a finding also noted both by American (8, 20) and English (9) workers. The rise in the actual number of blood cultures drawn likely reflects the general awareness that certain groups of patients are at particular risk of acquiring bacteremia and also the now generally practiced routine of obtaining a blood culture from seriously ill patients regardless of age (8). Interestingly there was little difference in the *ratio* of positive cultures to total cultures taken (9.69% vs. 9.79%), while the number of *patients* with bacteremia rose 91 percent (from 79 patients in 1960 to 151 patients in 1970). Accordingly, bacteremia at this institution rose from 5.63 per 1,000 admissions (1960) to 9.75 per 1,000 (1970) in the span of a decade, a figure that is very close to the frequency of all bacteremias in American hospitals projected as 10/1,000 admissions by Martin in 1969 (10).

It should be pointed out here that blood cultures that contained only *S. epidermidis, Bacillus* sp. or *Corynebacterium* sp. are not included in Table 1-I or in the calculations of frequencies below. This arbitrary decision was necessitated by the difficulty in differentiating between contaminating and significant isolates and because several published reports (3, 22), used for comparison, also omitted such cultures. However, it should be kept in mind that such organisms have been repeatedly cited in the literature as etiologic agents of endocarditis and of septicemia (24, 25, 26).

This increase in the overall rate of bacteremia, similar to findings elsewhere, is accounted for by the rise in incidence of gram-negative bacteremia. As shown in Table 1-I, there was practically no change in the frequency of gram-positive bacteremia from 1960 to 1970 (2.42/1,000 vs. 2.45/1,000 admissions) but bacteremia due to gram-negative bacilli increased 133 percent in the same period, i.e. from 2.71/1,000 to 6.33/1,000 admissions. In contrast, the incidence of gram-negative bacteremia in 1966 at the University of Minnesota Medical Center was 8.1/1,000 admissions (8); at a large southern hospital in 1965 it was 5.1/1,000 (20), and at Peter Bent Brigham Hospital in 1969 it reached 10.7 per 1,000 admissions (16), the highest incidence yet reported.

Both in 1960 and in 1970, *Escherichia coli* was the single species most frequently isolated from patients' bloodstream at The Jewish Hospital of St. Louis, as was the case in a number of other published series (5, 8, 15, 16). *E. coli* was isolated from 25.3 percent of bacteremic patients in 1960 and from 24.5 percent in 1970. *Klebsiella pneumoniae* isolations increased from 6.3 percent in 1960 to 11.9 percent in 1970, again consistent with findings in other series. The highest increases were shown by *Pseudomonas* (from 1.2% to 7.3%) and *Bacteroides* (1.2% to 6.6%) bacteremias. Thus, in 1970, *Bacteroides* bacteremia represented 10 percent of all gram-negative bacteremias at this institution.

The incidence of *Serratia* and *Enterobacter* bacteremia at The Jewish Hospital of St. Louis in 1970 (Table 1-I) was 5.2 percent, somewhat lower than the frequencies reported by other investigators (3, 8, 20).

The relative ranking and frequency of gram-negative organisms in bacteremia was determined from combined reports of 3,200 cases by McCabe (23) as follows: E. coli (37%), *Klebsiella-Enterobacter-Serratia* (20%), *Pseudomonas aeruginosa* (17%), *Proteus spp.* (11%). The ranking of these organisms for 1970 in Table 1-I (*E. coli*: 24.5%, *Klebsiella-Enterobacter-Serratia*: 17.1%, *P. aeruginosa*: 7.3%) is the same for the first three but *Bacteroides* is fourth in frequency, its incidence (6.6%) being higher than that of *Proteus* (5.2%). This is likely due to differences in anaerobic methodology employed in various laboratories and likely also to the selection of patients admitted to various hospitals. Washington (22), for the period of 1968 to 1970, reported Bacteroidaceae isolated from 13.8 percent of bacteremic patients at the Mayo Clinic, while in Dalton's series (20), over a 15-year period, Bacteroidaceae represented only 0.5 percent of etiologic agents of bacteremia. In a more recent series reported by Myerowitz *et al.* (16) Bacteroidaceae were isolated from 1.3 percent of bacteremic patients.

In contrast to gram-negative bacteremias, *Staphylococcus aureus* bloodstream infections declined from 12.6 percent to 6.6 percent, but *Streptococcus pyogenes*, group A infections increased from 1.2 percent to 4.6 percent (Table 1-I). A significant increase in the number of patients and deaths from hemolytic streptococcal bacteremia from 1955 on was also noted by Finland (3) at the Boston City Hospital.

There was a striking increase in the recovery of more than one species of bacteria from patients with bacteremia (polymicrobial infections), from 3.8 percent (1960) to 7.3 percent (1970) of all bloodstream infections (Table 1-I). Of the 11 polymicrobial infections seen in 1970, there were 5 patients with a combination of 2 gram-negative bacilli, 3 patients with a gram-negative and a gram-positive organism, and 3 patients who had three organisms isolated simultaneously from their blood cultures (Table 1-I). The increase in multiple-species bacteremia has also been documented by other reports (8); according to Hermans and Washington (21) and Washington (22), at least 6 percent of bacteremic patients have polymicrobial infection.

Less common bacterial species encountered in bacteremia at The Jewish Hospital of St. Louis (Table 1-I) and in other series (2, 3, 8, 17, 20, 21, 22, 26) include *Citrobacter, Providencia, Aeromonas, Acinetobacter* (Mima-Herellea), *Salmonella, Listeria, Clostridium,* and anaerobic streptococci, as well as *Yersinia* (27), *Edwardsiella* (27), *Actinobacillus, Vibrio fetus* (28), *Erwinia* and *Enterobacter agglomerans* (29), and *Bacillus cereus* (26).*

Problems in Search of Solution

The data presented above clearly indicate the magnitude of the bacteremia problem and also points to the numerous difficulties to be overcome before a reversal of the steady rise in frequency of bacteremia can be effected.

The use of effective antibiotics in serious life-threatening infections will obviously continue (3) and the selective pressure they will exert will undoubtedly persist. Intensified educational efforts directed toward reducing the indiscriminate application of large doses of antimicrobials used without the benefit of appropriate susceptibility tests and often employed, without justification, in trivial illnesses, have not been notably successful.

Aging of the hospital population is an inexorable process, as

---

* For a detailed discussion of unusual agents of bacteremia, see Chapter 4.

is the continuing application and further development of ever more sophisticated and radical life-lengthening procedures, i.e. radio- and immunotherapy, surgical procedures, transplantation, etc., with their attendant risks. Thus, efforts for the amelioration and reversal of the rising trend of bacteremia must be directed toward other factors.

Among these, the role of the clinical microbiology laboratory is a pivotal one that bears careful scrutiny. It is generally agreed that bacteremia is a precise diagnosis based upon blood culture (2), obtained *before* antibiotics are administered. Blood cultures are necessary to (a) determine whether the patient indeed has bacteremia, (b) establish the identity of the infecting organism and (c) allow the performance of antibiotic susceptibility tests on the isolates. It is also obvious that the conventional methods of blood culture and susceptibility testing, as practiced currently, are less than ideal in terms of accomplishing rapid detection, recovery, identification and antibiotic susceptibility determinations of the infecting organism.

The delay, ranging from 24 to 72 hours (and sometimes even longer) experienced in the delivery of precise, therapeutically useful laboratory information poses a significant problem in the treatment of bacteremia. Improvements in and innovations of methods for optimal and early detection, and for rapid recovery, identification, and susceptibility tests of the infecting organism are needed to allow for rational therapy. Early detection of growth by radiometric methods, and the use of non-cultural technics, such as gas chromatography for detection of metabolites from bacterial growth (see Chapter 6), as well as the *Limulus polyphemus* (horseshoe crab) assay (30, 31) for the detection of endotoxins of gram-negative organisms, need to be further explored to determine their value in the detection of bacteremia.

The reduction of bacteremia rates also depends on better and more stringent methods for the control and elimination of external sources of infection (*common-source* outbreaks) as well as the careful isolation and handling of the infected patient, so that his infection (contact transfer) does not spread to other, highly susceptible patients.

Last, but not least, there is need for gathering and effectively disseminating information about current blood culture practices and the evaluation of their efficacy, techniques for early detection of bacteremia, the involvement and significance of so-called unusual, anaerobic and fastidious organisms in bacteremia, and the occurrence and possible control of common-source outbreaks due to such products as contaminated intravenous fluids, or to blood or platelet transfusions. Much of our present knowledge concerning these problems is elaborated in the ensuing chapters.

REFERENCES

1. Finland, M.; Jones, W. F., and Barnes, M. W.: Occurrence of serious bacterial infections since introduction of antibacterial agents. *JAMA, 170*:2188, 1959.
2. Brumfitt, W., and Leigh, D. A.: Gram-negative septicaemia. *Proc R Soc Med, 62*:1239, 1969.
3. Finland, M.: Changing ecology of bacterial infections as related to antibacterial therapy. *J Infect Dis, 122*:419, 1970.
4. Waisbren, B.: Bacteremia due to gram-negative bacilli other than the *Salmonella*: A clinical and therapeutic study. *Arch Intern Med, 88*:467, 1951.
5. McCabe, W. R., and Jackson, G. G.: Gram-negative bacteremia. *Arch Intern Med, 110*:847, 1962.
6. Altemeier, W. A.; Todd, J. C., and Inge, W. W.: Gram-negative septicemia: A growing threat. *Ann Surg, 166*:530, 1967.
7. Fried, M. A., and Vosti, K. L.: The importance of underlying disease in patients with gram-negative bacteremia. *Arch Intern Med, 121*:418, 1968.
8. DuPont, H. L., and Spink, W. W.: Infections due to Gram-negative organisms: An analysis of 860 patients with bacteremia at the University of Minnesota Medical Center, 1958-1966. *Medicine, 48*:307, 1969.
9. Crowley, N.: Some bacteraemias encountered in hospital practice. *J Clin Pathol, 23*:166, 1970.
10. Martin, C. M.: A national bacteremia registry. *J Infect Dis, 120*:495, 1969.
11. Shallard, M. A., and Williams, A. L.: A study of the carriage of gram-negative bacilli by newborn babies in hospital. *Med J Aust, 1*:540, 1965.
12. Watt, P. J., and Okubadejo, O. A.: Changes in incidence and aetiology of bacteraemia arising in hospital practice. *Br Med J, 1*:210, 1967.
13. Lepper, M. H.; Moulton, B.; Dowling, H. F.; Jackson, G. G., and Kofman, S.: Epidemiology of erythromycin-resistant staphylococci

in a hospital population—effect on therapeutic activity of erythromycin. *In* Antibiotics Annual 1953-54, Welch, H., and Marti-Ibanez, F., eds. New York, Medical Encyclopedia, Inc., 1953.

14. Pollack, M.; Nieman, R. E.; Reinhardt, J. A.; Charache, P.; Jett, M. P., and Hardy, P. H.: Factors influencing colonisation and antibiotic-resistance patterns of gram-negative bacteria in hospital patients. *Lancet, II*:668, 1972.

15. McHenry, M. C.; Martin, W. J., and Wellman, W. E.: Bacteremia due to gram-negative bacilli. *Ann Intern Med, 56*:207, 1962.

16. Myerowitz, R. L.; Mederios, A. A., and O'Brien, T. F.: Recent experience with bacillemia due to gram-negative organisms. *J Infect Dis, 124*:239, 1971.

17. Martin, W. J., and McHenry, M. C.: Bacteremia due to gram-negative bacilli. *Journal-Lancet, 84*:385, 1964.

18. Parker, M. T.: Causes and prevention of sepsis due to gram-negative bacteria: Ecology of the infecting organisms. *Proc R Soc Med, 64*:979, 1971.

19. Bassett, D. J. C.: Causes and prevention of sepsis due to gram-negative bacteria: Common-source outbreaks. *Proc R Soc Med, 64*:980, 1971.

20. Dalton, H. P., and Allison, M. J.: Etiology of bacteremia. *Appl Microbiol, 15*:808, 1967.

21. Hermans, P. E., and Washington, J. A.: Polymicrobial bacteremia. *Ann Intern Med, 73*:387, 1970.

22. Washington, J. A.: Comparison of two commercially available media for detection of bacteremia. *Appl Microbiol, 22*:604, 1971.

23. McCabe, W. R.: Gram-negative bacteremia: A physician's overview. *In*: Gram-negative sepsis, Sanford, J. P., ed. New York, Medcom, 1971.

24. Allison, M. J.; Gerszten, E., and Dalton, H. P.: Bacterial endocarditis. *South Med J, 60*:129, 1967.

25. Wittler, R. G.; Malizia, W. F.; Kramer, P. E.; Ruckett, J. D.; Pritchard, H. N., and Baker, H. J.: Isolation of a corynebacterium and its transitional forms from a case of S.B.E. treated with antibiotics. *J Gen Microbiol, 23*:315, 1960.

26. Leffert, H. L.; Baptist, J. N., and Gidez, L. I.: Meningitis and bacteremia after ventriculoatrial shunt-revision: Isolation of a lecithinase-producing *Bacillus cereus. J Infect Dis, 122*:547, 1970.

27. Sonnenwirth, A. C.: Bacteremia with and without meningitis due to *Yersinia enterocolitica, Edwardsiella tarda, Comamonas terrigena,* and *Pseudomonas maltophilia. Ann NY Acad Sci, 174*(Art. 2):488, 1970.

28. Bokkenheuser, V.: Vibrio fetus infection in man. I. Ten new cases and some epidemiologic observations. *Am J Epidemiol, 91*:400, 1970.

29. Ewing, W. H., and Fife, M. A.: *Enterobacter agglomerans.* Atlanta, Center for Disease Control, 1971.
30. Levin, J.; Margolis, S., and Bell, W. R.: Gram-negative sepsis: Detection of endotoxemia with the Limulus test. *Ann Intern Med,* 76:1, 1972.
31. Sonnenwirth, A. C.; Yin, E. T.; Sarmiento, E. M., and Wessler, S.: Bacteroidaceae endotoxin detection by Limulus assay. *Am J Clin Nutr,* 25:1452, 1972.

CHAPTER 2

CONTEMPORARY BLOOD CULTURE PRACTICES

RAYMOND C. BARTLETT, M.D.

INTRODUCTION

To THOSE WHO HAVE compared blood culture practices in various clinical laboratories, more variation may have been apparent in procedure and materials used than in any other commonly performed diagnostic microbiologic procedure. The basis for this chapter is a review of blood culture practices in twenty-one proficient clinical laboratories directed by eminent microbiologists and clinical pathologists (Figure 2-1). Recently many exciting alternatives to conventional methods for isolation and identification of bacteria in patients with bacteremia have

Laboratory	Director
Sacramento Medical Center	Arthur Barry
Hartford Hospital	Raymond Bartlett
University of Illinois	Leon LeBeau
Gottlieb Hospital	Esther Cheatle
Berkshire Medical Center	George Douglas
Columbia University	Paul Ellner
Wadsworth VA Hospital	Maurice White
Cleveland Clinic	Thomas Gavan
Springfield Hospital Medical Center	Dieter Groschel
Massachusetts General Hospital	Lawrence Kunz
University of Minnesota	John Matsen
Thomas Jefferson University Hospital	Eileen Randall
Long Beach Memorial Hospital	James Reynolds
St. Joseph's Hospital	Richard Rosner
University of Washington	Fritz Schoenknecht
Delaware Hospital	Elvyn Scott
Passavent Memorial Hospital	Herbert Sommers
Jewish Hospital, St. Louis	Alex Sonnenwirth
University of Connecticut	Richard Tilton
Yale Medical Center	Alex von Graevenitz
Mayo Clinic	John Washington

Figure 2-1. Laboratories and directors participating in blood culture survey, April, 1971.

appeared. The potential value of gas chromatography applied both to patient serum and culture media has stimulated considerable interest (1). Acceleration of isolation has been claimed and refuted in studies of the use of radioactive substrates (2, 3). A number of investigators and manufacturers have promoted the use of filtration collection and culture systems (4, 5). Ten percent sucrose for isolation of cell wall deficient forms, and the anticoagulant sodium polyanethol sulfonate (SPS) have received acclaim (6, 7, 8). The participants in this survey were queried on all of these procedures. Little practical interest or experience was expressed with the exception of the addition of SPS. This report is made with the sobering recognition that existing blood culture technique will likely continue to predominate for many years. Reference will be made to relevant published information as each aspect of the subject is discussed.

Laboratory Workloads

The hospitals represented ranged considerably in size from one hundred twenty beds to fourteen hundred beds. There was a large difference in the number of blood cultures collected per year per bed (Fig. 2-2). Hartford Hospital fell close to the middle of the distribution. Three institutions exceeding fifteen blood culture collections per year per bed were major medical school affiliated teaching hospitals. Those with less than five blood culture collections per year per bed included hospitals with minor teaching affiliations or no specific undergraduate medical affiliations. A tenfold range of distribution in beds per fulltime microbiology laboratory worker was observed. Our hospital fell near the center of the distribution. Values below 20 were associated with large major teaching hospitals and values exceeding 70 were found in hospitals with minor or no undergraduate teaching affiliation. A similar tenfold range or distribution was observed for numbers of microbiologic specimens processed per fulltime worker. Here again, our laboratory fell near the mean. High and low volumes were correlated with extent of major medical teaching commitments. Of 86 laboratories in which specimen volumes in bacteriology were surveyed and reported elsewhere (9), 52 handled less than four thousand five hundred specimens per year per worker and 34 exceeded this amount. This striking range in effort as well as cost expended was reflected in the range of blood culture collections processed per fulltime worker in the 21 laboratories included in this survey. The range correlates as before with extent of educational involvement within the institution but in addition, correlates with the numbers of subcultures performed. The lowest volume of two thousand cultures per worker per year was reported by the only laboratory which routinely performed four subcultures on all collections. The laboratory reporting fifteen thousand collections per worker per year did not routinely perform subcultures. The matter of subculture will be explored in greater depth later.

Numbers and Frequency of Collections

Unlike most other laboratory specimens, physicians are responsible for larger numbers of blood culture collections than other groups of personnel. Whether physicians collect cultures or order them to be collected by others, many clinical microbiologists have questioned whether some limit should be imposed on the number of collections and the time interval between collections. It has been our practice to limit collections to four per day. If additional cultures are requested, the nursing unit is informed that the physician must consult with the microbiologist before additional collections will be made. On rare occasions, physicians will personally collect up to a dozen blood cultures more or less simultaneously and submit them to the laboratory. One has no choice but to process these under such conditions. None of the other laboratories in the survey indicated that they could control the number of cultures requested by physicians. Only four indicated that they could control the interval between collections. Thirteen of the twenty-one respondents did not even feel that they were in a position to make recommendations for the number of cultures or the interval of time between collections. Of those who have been in the practice of making such recommendations, most suggested three per day with a wide distribution of recommended intervals. In a

Figure 2-2. Results of blood culture survey; twenty-one laboratories.

1) Beds

XXX	XXXXXX XXXXX	XX XX X	XXX		X
100	300 500	700	900	1100	1300

2) Blood culture collections/year/bed

```
            X       X
            X       X                           X
  X XXXXXXX XXXⓍ    XX              X            X
  0       5         10             15           20
```

3) Beds/full time worker (Microbiol.)

```
  X XXX      XX X    XⓍX XXXXX    XXX      XX        XX
 10          30      50           70               100
```

4) Microbiol. Spec./full time worker (thousands/year)

```
  X       XXXXX XXXXXXXXⓍ  XXX   XX          X      X
  1     2      3      4    5     6     7     8      9      10
```

5) Blood culture collections processed/full time worker; thousands/year

```
XXXXXXXXX X              XXX   ⓍXX X  X                         X
2         4      6              8      10          12      14
```

6) Method of collection

	Routine	Stat	Night
Microbiol. personnel	3	3	1
Lab technicians	4	3	4
Special collectors	9	7	3
Physicians	12	15	16

7) Ability to control: *number* of collections/day

YES 1 NO 20

interval between collections
YES 4 NO 17

8) Limits established or recommended

Number

None	13	5 minutes	1
3/day	4	30 minutes	2
4/day	1	1 hour	1
3-6/day	1	2 hours	1
6/day	1	3 hours	1
12/day	1	4 hours	1

9) Skin preparation *actually in use*

tincture iodine and alcohol	11
alcohol	3
Betadine and alcohol	3
Betadine	1
soap water, Betadine	1
Phisohex, iodine, alcohol	1
unknown	1

10) Blood cultures collected separate from other laboratory specimens

YES   16   NO   4

11) Amount collected   Dilution

10 ml	15	1:10	13
1 ml	1 (peds)	1:15	1
12 ml	2	1:20	3
8 ml	1		
15 ml	1		

12) Syringe 15; transfer set 5

13) Commercial media   15
    Lab prepared media   6

14) Volume

Volume	50	10
	100	6
	140	1
	?	4

15) Broth only   16
    with pour plate   3
    with Castaneda   2

16) Media used

T Soy	11
Thio	6
Thiol	6
Brucella	3
Columbia	3
BHI	2
TSY	1
Dext-PO$_4$	1

17) Capneic Incubation 15

18) Anaerobic method

Thio-Thiol	12
0.1% agar	3
E med.	2
anaerobic incub.	
evac. bottle	3
jar	2
subculture anaer. plate	1
none	1

19) SPS added 15
   in medium 9
   in transport 3

20) Penicillinase added
   on request 10
   not used 10

21) Days of Incubation

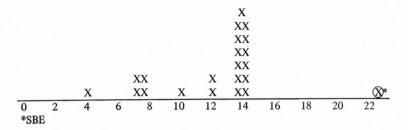

*SBE

22) Number and Day of Subcultures (no obvious growth)

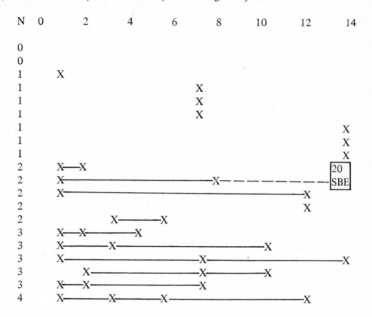

23) Subculture procedure

based on Gram stain	2
Plates: Chocolate	19
BAP	13
BHI	1
DOC	1
Kan agar	1
Anaerobic plates	12
Broth: thio	6
chopped meat	1

24) Perform direct disc susceptibility test?

YES   16   NO   4

25) Adjust inoculum density in direct test?

YES   6   NO   10

26) Confirm susceptibility with standard procedure

YES   14   NO   2

27) Criteria for performance of broth dilution
    and serum inhibition tests

done on request	7
consult infectious dis. only	5
SBE cases only	3
Separate lab	3
all positive cultures	2
Staph, Strep cases	2
never done	1

28) Percent cultures probably contaminated

unknown	1	5%	4	> 25%	3
1%	4	10%	2		
2%	4	20%	3		

    (Staph epidermidis; Corynebacterium sp.)

29) Percent positive cultures

unknown	1
2%	1
5%	1
6-7%	3
8-10%	5
12-14%	5
15-17%	2
>20%	1

30) Percent positive isolates mixed but probably
    not contamination

unknown	1
<1%	12
3%	1
6%	1
10%	2

31) Report *anything* isolated

YES	18	NO	2

32) When would you *not* report an isolate

Never	12
Obvious contamination on pour plate	2
Obvious lab contaminant	3
Anaerobe from E medium after 14 days	1
1 of 3 cultures showing Corynebacterium	1
or Staph epidermidis	

33) Do you ever qualify report with
"Possible" or Probable Contamination"

YES   12   NO   7

34) Culture of blood bank blood from transfusion
reactions and routine screening

Same as others	5
Same as others but also 4°-22°C.	3
AABB procedure	4
NIH procedure	1
Misc. Thio, BAP, aerobic, anaerobic,	6
different temperatures	

35) Hypertonic medium used?

YES, worthwhile	2
YES, not worthwhile	1
YES, special cases	3
NO	9

36) Pre-reduced medium?

YES	2
NEXT YEAR	4
NO	9

37) Filtration procedures used?

YES	0
"Mickey Mouse"	7
Contamination problems	1
H. flu wouldn't grow	1
Adjunct in selected cases	1

38) Isotopic gas procedure?

could not corroborate claims   1

39)   Gas chromatography

planning study soon   1

study of two hundred six cases of bacterial endocarditis, over a sixteen year period, Werner *et al.* reported that 97 percent of blood cultures were positive when no previous antibiotics had been given (10). Ninety-one percent were positive when the patient had received previous antimicrobial therapy. In this study, no case without previous antimicrobial therapy required more than three blood cultures to establish the etiologic agent. When antibiotics had been given, no more than seven cultures were required.

Little information is available to indicate the number of blood cultures that are required to establish the etiologic agent in other types of bacteremias. We conducted a study of 59 culture positive septicemias to determine the numbers of blood cultures that were required to identify the infecting organism. No attempt was made to separate those patients who were and were not receiving antibiotics during the period in which blood cultures were collected. There were 14 (24%) septicemias in which the first culture failed to reveal the infecting agent. On the other hand, in 76 percent, the first culture was positive. In 7 instances (12%), the agent failed to appear in either the first or second culture. Only 2 septicemias occurred (3%) in which the infecting agent was not demonstrated in one of the first three cultures collected. In no instance were more than four cultures required to demonstrate the infecting organism (Fig. 2-3).

It is generally accepted that the bacteremia of bacterial endocarditis is a constant process. Some have suggested that the collection of 40 cc represents a sufficient sample of blood to assure isolation of the infecting agent. For practical purposes, this is usually done in divided collections. Potential contamination of a single large volume collection will create more confusion than contamination of one of several divided collections. There is no basis for establishing an interval between divided collections. This should be dictated by practicality. In septicemia

SEPTICEMIA AND FREQUENCY OF POSITIVE BLOOD CULTURES

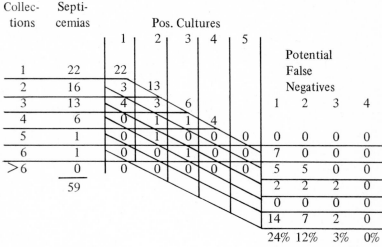

Figure 2-3. Evaluation of 59 culture positive septicemias for minimum number of collections required to isolate bacterial agents with confidence.

from other sources such as urinary tract infection, pneumonia, etc., it has been demonstrated that bacterial showers occur sporadically and are associated with chills and fever. An attempt is usually made to collect blood cultures when these symptoms appear. In conclusion, it could be recommended that a maximum of four blood cultures be collected during any twenty-four hour period for the diagnosis of bacterial endocarditis or other types of septicemia. Double this number seems justified if the patient has received antibiotics during the previous forty-eight hours. A minimum interval of one hour between collections seems the practical limitation in cases of subacute bacterial endocarditis. In other types of septicemia, including acute endocarditis caused by *Staphylococcus aureus* or various Enterobacteriaceae, the collection should be correlated with the appearance of symptoms. Occasionally a fairly obvious case of subacute bacterial endocarditis will prompt rapid collection of cultures to allow immediate antibiotic therapy. There is no evidence that one or two hours of delay in therapy will alter the course of subacute bacterial endocarditis. During this time, the necessary cultures can be conveniently collected. In other types of bacteremia, especially those associated with gram negative sepsis, rapid initiation of therapy is important. Under these conditions, the collection of four cultures in two separate venipunctures may be performed immediately. The volume of blood and number of containers inoculated will be discussed below. For purposes of this discussion, a collection is considered a 10 ml sample divided into two separate containers for aerobic and anaerobic culture.

Collection

Tincture of iodine followed by alcohol was the commonest form of skin preparation found in this survey (Fig. 2-2). No correlation was found between the method of skin preparation and the estimated level of contamination. It is doubtful that any form of skin decontamination which can be applied only for a fraction of a minute will significantly reduce the bacterial flora of the deeper layers of the skin. The major effect is that of mechanical removal of superficial soil and bacteria, regardless of the solution used. It is our view that the use of two solutions assures a somewhat more thorough cleansing process than one. It is unfortunate that most technicians disinfect with the dominant side hand, but palpate for the vein with the other. Since palpation is inevitable, contact of these disinfectants with the same fingers that are used for palpation would significantly reduce this source of bacterial contamination.

Effect of Volume, Dilution and Additives

The only anticoagulant found to be used in this survey was sodium polyanethol sulfonate, SPS, which was incorporated in the transport tube of three of the responding laboratories and used in the culture medium of nine others. Attention has been drawn to the toxic effects of citrate and other anticoagulants (11). The anticomplementary, antiphagocytic and antibiotic neutralizing properties, and the lack of toxicity, of SPS should exclude the use of any other anticoagulant (11).

Several reports have clearly documented the increased yield of positive cultures from body fluids containing various penicillins following the addition of penicillinase (12, 13). In spite of this, half of the respondents indicated that penicillinase was not used at all; the other half used it only when specifically requested. Although we have found penicillinase solutions extremely stable for months at refrigerator temperatures, contamination is a significant problem and periodic cultures should be performed to avoid introducing spurious bacteria (14).

Ellner (11) demonstrated a reduction in contamination from 8 percent to 2 percent with a change from inoculation of open to closed flasks. In spite of the appearance of transfer sets for convenient inoculation of pre-evacuated blood culture bottles, most of the respondents in this survey continue to use syringes. The majority collected 10 ml of blood which was divided into two culture containers. This results in the commonly recommended one to ten dilution if each of the vessels contains 50 ml of medium. Most workers believe that collection of less than 10 ml of blood reduces the probability of a positive culture. Werner *et al.* (10) drew attention to this factor in regard to a report by Belli and Waisbren (15) in which an incidence of only 53 percent positive cultures in patients with bacterial endocarditis was found. This was based on a system in which only five ml of blood had been collected. Werner *et al.* also reported data from pour plates used in the cultures of patients in their study. In several cases, no colonies appeared in pour plates. In half, less than thirty colonies per ml were found. Recently, a compact blood collecting tube containing twenty ml of culture medium has become available commercially. Only 2 ml of blood is inoculated. Unpublished comparative studies* between this technique and one in which five ml of blood was sampled and cultured aerobically have demonstrated comparable efficiency in recovering bacteria in 248 instances of septicemia. It is possible that the comparable yield obtained with the smaller sample of blood is a reflection of (a) greater enrichment; (b) low Eh, resulting partially from the incorporation of agar and cysteine; (c) the addition of sodium polyanethol sulfonate, and of penicillinase. More extensive trials will be required to dis-

---

* Becton-Dickinson, Rutherford, New Jersey.

place the widely held conviction that a 10 ml sample will produce a higher percentage of positive cultures.

Certain commercial blood culture units containing twenty-five to thirty ml of broth result in a lower dilution ratio. Reports of Mackie and Finkelstein (16, 17) and of others (18, 19, 20) demonstrated many years ago that the natural inhibitory titer of serum would effectively prevent growth of bacteria in 1:10 and frequently greater dilutions. Indeed, titers in the range of 1:1,600 were described for inhibition of the growth of *Salmonella typhi* in the presence of the patient's own serum. This is the basis for the time-honored recommendation that clots be cultured following separation of serum in patients suspected of typhoid fever. Review of these publications convinces one that the dilution ratio should be considerably higher than one to ten and certainly should not be reduced.

Media in Use

Most of the respondents utilized only broth culture media. The use of pour plates or Castaneda bottles which provide enumeration of colonies finds little support and has been abandoned in most laboratories. The claim that enumeration assists in identifying contamination is not consistent with Werner's data (10) in which none to over one hundred colonies per ml were found. Some suggest that it provides early identification of mixed cultures which represent probable contamination. As will be discussed below, there is reason to believe that the incidence of mixed bacteremias is higher than has been appreciated. Other attributes include: earlier identification by observation of types of hemolysis around streptococci; automatic provision of subculture without entering the bottle. Most workers believe that subculture to fresh medium free of the inhibitory action of serum, antibiotics, and metaboiltes is preferable.

Tryptic digest of casein soy broth was the commonest medium used and was closely followed by thioglycollate and Thiol®* medium. Most of the respondents used capneic incubation for these media. Only one of the respondents did not use some

---

* Thiol is a registered product of Difco Laboratories, Detroit, Michigan.

specific method for isolation of anaerobes (Fig. 2-2). Felner and Dowell (26) reported a 14 percent incidence of isolation of anaerobes from one thousand forty-six reported cases of bacterial endocarditis. We observed an increase from one to thirty-one in the annual number of cases of *Bacteroides* bacteremia following the routine introduction of anaerobic cultures of blood. Two of the respondents used a specifically prereduced medium. Some confusion has resulted from the presence of killed rumen bacteria which appear in gram stains prepared from such media.

Duration of Incubation and Subculture

A trend toward reduction in the duration of incubation has occurred in recent years. Most of the respondents in this survey incubated cultures for fourteen days. Four reported an incubation period of only seven days. This trend is the result of reports by Effersoe in 1967 (21) and Ellner (11) who reported not one positive culture after the fifth day in a review of forty thousand specimens. Older literature containing reports of several weeks of incubation for isolation of *Salmonella* and *Brucella* have had a major influence on traditional practice (22, 23, 24).

Conservatives still point to sporadic isolates of *Streptococcus viridans* between one and two weeks in patients with endocarditis. Recently, we have observed two patients with delayed isolation of anaerobes: the first was a case of endometritis from which a *Peptostreptococcus* was isolated after seven days, while the other occurred in a patient with an abdominal abscess in which *Bacteroides fragilis* was isolated from the abscess but blood cultures required more than one week to become positive for the same organism. In neither of these cases had antibiotics been given prior to the collection of cultures. In a series of five hundred positive blood cultures in our laboratory, 12 percent became positive after seven days. Seven percent of these could have been explained by contamination but the remaining 5 percent were considered clinically significant. Two of the respondents did not routinely subculture blood cultures in the absence of apparent growth. We have frequently observed blood cultures which show no evidence of growth but upon subculture, demonstrate *Neisseria gonorrhoeae, Haemophilus influenzae,* or

Streptococcus pneumoniae. A diverse pattern of subculture practice was reported by the respondents. It is difficult to build an academic case for any particular number or schedule of subcultures. If any consensus can be derived from the results of the survey (Fig. 2-2) it would appear to be two subcultures, the first at twenty-four hours and the second at seven days. The added expense of a third subculture at the end of fourteen days on bottles not showing apparent growth seems unjustified.

Most of the respondents indicated that subcultures were made to chocolate agar but there was no clear majority on use of other types of media. Two indicated that the choice of media was based entirely on the results of gram stain. Ellner (25) has recently described a system involving centrifugation, and inoculation of substrates for rapid identification of organism growth in blood culture bottles.

Contamination, Number of Positive Cultures and Mixed Cultures

In this survey a wide range of values was given for the probable numbers of contaminated blood cultures. Most responses fell in the range of 1 to 5 percent, but three respondents indicated that over 25 percent of their cultures appeared to be contaminated. It is difficult to establish criteria which clearly distinguish contamination from bacteremia. Most workers define this condition as the isolation of *Corynebacterium, Propionibacterium, Staphylococcus epidermidis* and *Bacillus* species from patients who do not demonstrate factors which would predispose them to infection with these organisms, i.e. intraventricular shunts cardiovascular and prosthetic valve surgery. In a study of 161 consecutive positive blood cultures in our laboratory, 25 percent demonstrated isolation of these species of bacteria. As previously indicated, the method of skin preparation demonstrated no correlation with the estimates of contamination. Furthermore, there was no correlation with the numbers of subcultures.

The percentage of positive blood cultures fell between 6 and 15 percent for most of the participating laboratories. There was no correlation between this percentage, the numbers of blood cultures per bed, incidence of suspected contamination or number of subcultures performed (Fig. 2-2).

Respondents indicated that less than 1 percent of clinically significant blood cultures contained more than one kind of organism. The finding of anaerobes mixed with aerobes in 24 percent of a series of bacterial endocarditis cases studied by Fellner and Dowell was referred to above (26). Hochstein (27) using an elaborate system involving four separate media, each subcultured on four separate occasions, reported an incidence for mixed blood cultures of 8 percent. McCabe and Jackson indicated that 10 percent of gram negative septicemias were mixed (28). Of the series of 59 septicemias observed in this hospital, six (10%) contained more than one bacterial species. These reports contrasted with the results of this survey suggest that more effort should be expended on identification of mixed positive blood cultures. We have observed a case of bacterial endocarditis from which two strains of enterococcus were isolated, with significantly different levels of susceptibility to penicillin.

Reporting

Eighteen of the respondents indicated that they would report anything that was isolated from a blood culture. Twelve stated that they would qualify the report with "possible" or "probable contamination." In this era of increasing frequency of opportunistic infection, no microorganism can be so well categorized as a contaminant that the report can be rendered as *sterile* without some clinical investigation. *Staphylococcus epidermidis, Corynebacterium,* or *Propionibacterium* species isolated from only one of several blood cultures are almost certainly contaminants but the knowledgeable clinical microbiologist should establish whether predisposing factors such as ventricular shunts or evidence of endocarditis exist before labeling such a culture as contaminated. It was apparent from the survey that few workers have the time, or feel that it is their prerogative to make a distinction between isolates of this type which may be clinically significant and those which are not. The reporting of the sporadic isolation of these species from blood culture collections occasionally may result in diagnostic confusion including an erroneous diagnosis of bacteremia resulting in misdirected antimicrobial therapy. The best compromise would be to qualify reports of the isolation of these particular species from only one of two or more blood cultures stating that possible or probable contamination has occurred.

Antimicrobial Susceptibility Testing

Direct susceptibility tests were performed from positive blood cultures by most of the respondents without standardization of the inoculum density. In most cases, these results were confirmed by the standardized Kirby-Bauer procedure (29).

The laboratory directors participating in the survey were asked about their criteria for performing quantitative antimicrobial susceptibility and serum inhibition titers. A variety of circumstances were reported to affect the availability of these procedures. Only one indicated that these tests were not performed.

Culture of Blood Bank Blood

A variety of techniques were used for the culture of blood bank blood. Most of these incorporated features of the recommended procedures of the American Association of Blood Banks (30). This calls for incubation at several temperatures ranging from 18° C to 37° C with subculture on the third to the fifth day.

CONCLUDING REMARKS

A wide variety of practices for the processing of blood cultures were found in a survey of 21 prominent clinical microbiology laboratories. Except for the failure of one laboratory to subculture at all and the omission by another of a method for isolation of anaerobes, each laboratory's approach would appear to be in accord with available knowledge of the isolation of microorganisms from bacteremic patients.

In this period of growing public concern over cost of medical care, attention should be drawn to the remarkable differences in numbers of blood cultures processed per worker. Since the major cost involved in blood culture procedures is labor, it could be estimated that the laboratory which processed only two thousand blood cultures per year per worker incurred four to five times the cost per specimen demonstrated by the majority of the laboratories in this survey. It has already been noted that this laboratory was providing services for an institution with major educational commitments. It was the only laboratory which routinely performed four subcultures on all specimens.

It is likely that third parties who must pay these costs will begin to base reimbursements on the minimum cost which appears consistent with either typical standards in clinical laboratories or the lowest standard which appears capable of providing the information required. A challenge to the uneconomical operations of many academically oriented centers is long overdue. Instead of incurring the largest volumes of clinical laboratory work at a greater per patient cost, using methods which exceed the standards of a cross-section of proficient laboratories, forces currently gathering momentum in our society will proscribe that such institutions control the numbers as well as minimum analytical standards for performance of clinical laboratory procedures, or be denied reimbursement. It seems imperative that more attention should be given to the cost benefit of increasing numbers of specimens and to the complexity of their analysis.

REFERENCES

1. Cherry, W. W., and Moss, C. W.: The role of gas chromatography in the clinical microbiology laboratory. *J Infect Dis, 119*:658, 1969.
2. Deland, F., and Wagner, H. N., Jr.: Automated radiometric detection of bacterial growth in blood cultures. *J Lab Clin Med, 75*:529, 1970.
3. Washington, J. A., and Yu, P. K.: Radiometric method for detection of bacteremia. *Appl Microbiol, 22*:100, 1971.
4. Kozub, W. R.; Kirkham, W. R.; Chatman, C. E., and Pribor, H. C.: A practical blood culturing method employing dilution and filtration. *Am J Clin Path, 52*:105, 1969.
5. Finegold, S. M.; White, M. L.; Ziment, I., and Winn, W. R.: Rapid diagnosis of bacteremia. *Appl Microbiol, 18*:458, 1969.
6. Rosner, R.: Comparison of a blood culture system containing liquoid and sucrose with systems containing either reagent alone. *Appl Microbiol, 19*:281, 1970.
7. Rosner, R.: Effect of various anticoagulants and no anticoagulant on

ability to isolate bacteria directly from parallel clinical blood specimens. *Am J Clin Path, 49*:216, 1968.

8. Traub, W. H., and Lawrence, B. L.: Anticomplementary, anticoagulatory, and serum protein precipitating activity of sodium polyanethol sulfonate. *Appl Microbiol, 20*:465, 1970.

9. Bartlett, R. C.; Carrington, G. O., and Mielert, C.: *Quality Control in Clinical Microbiology* (rev.). Chicago, American Society of Clinical Pathologists, 1968.

10. Werner, A. S.; Cobbs, C. G.; Kaye, D., and Hook, E. W.: Studies on the bacteremia of bacterial endocarditis. *JAMA, 202*:127, 1967.

11. Ellner, P. D.: System for inoculation of blood in the laboratory. *Appl Microbiol, 16*:1892, 1968.

12. Dowling, H. F., and Hirsh, H. L.: Use in cultures of body fluids obtained from patients under treatment with penicillin. *Am J Med Sci, 210*:756, 1945.

13. Carleton, J. C., and Hamburger, M.: Unmasking of false-negative blood cultures in patients receiving new penicillins. *JAMA, 186*:157, 1963.

14. Norden, C. W.: Pseudo-septicemia. *Ann Intern Med, 71*:789, 1969.

15. Belli, J., and Waisbren, B. A.: The number of blood cultures necessary to diagnose most cases of bacterial endocarditis. *Am J Med Sci, 232*:284, 1956.

16. Mackie, T. J., and Finkelstein, M. H.: The bactericidins of normal serum: their characters, occurrence in various animals and their susceptibility of different bacteria to their action. *J Lab Clin Med, 32*:1, 1932.

17. Mackie, T. J., and Finkelstein, M. H.: Natural bactericidal antibodies: observations on the bactericidal mechanism of normal serum. *J Hyg, 31*:35, 1931.

18. Miles, A. A., and Misra, S. S.: The estimation of the bactericidal power of the blood. *J Hyg, 38*:732, 1938.

19. Khairat, O.: The bactericidal power of the blood for the infecting organism in bacteremia. *J Path Bact, 58*:359, 1946.

20. Gerstung, R. B.: Nonspecific inhibition by serum and urine in the microbiologic assay of antibiotics. *J Lab Clin Med, 37*:575, 1951.

21. Effersoe, P.: The importance of the duration of incubation in the investigation of blood cultures. *Acta Path Microbiol Scand, 65*:129, 1965.

22. Pulvertaft, R. J.: The clinical interpretation of aids to diagnosis. *Lancet, 1*:821, 1930.

23. Shaw, A. B., and Mackay, A. F.: Factors influencing results of blood culture in enteric fever. *J Hyg, 49*:315, 1951.

24. Watson, K. C.: Isolation of *Salmonella typhi* from the bloodstream. *J Lab Clin Med, 46*:125, 1955.

25. Wasilauskas, B. L., and Ellner, P. D.: Presumptive identification of bacteria from blood cultures in four hours. *J Infect Dis, 124*:499, 1971.
26. Felner, J. M., and Dowell, V. R., Jr.: Anaerobic bacterial endocarditis. *N Engl J Med, 282*:1188, 1970.
27. Hochstein, H. D.; Kirkham, W. R., and Young, V. M.: Recovery of more than 1 organism in septicemias. *N Engl J Med, 273*:468, 1965.
28. McCabe, W. R., and Jackson, G. G.: Gram negative bacteremia I. Etiology and ecology. *Arch Intern Med, 110*:842, 1962.
29. Bauer, A. W.; Kirby, W. M.; Sherris, J. C., and Turck, M.: Antibiotic susceptibility testing by a standardized single disk method. *Am J Clin Path, 45*:493, 1966.
30. American Association of Blood Banks: *Technical methods and procedures,* Ed. 5. Chicago, 1970.

CHAPTER 3

EARLY DETECTION OF BACTEREMIA

SYDNEY M. FINEGOLD, M.D.

BLOOD CULTURES ARE relatively unique among laboratory tests inasmuch as they may provide both definitive clinical diagnosis and specific etiologic diagnosis. Further underlining the importance of early detection of bacteremia are the facts that 1) mortality is still significant in patients with sepsis (20-25% overall and 60-80% when shock is present) and that 2) the sooner a septic patient is treated with the appropriate antimicrobial the more likely he is to recover.

Techniques for blood culture in general use presently are unsatisfactory in several respects:

1. Growth is relatively slow.

2. Broth blood cultures must be subcultured to solid media to obtain surface colonies for observation of colonial morphology and for subsequent identification procedures. Recognition of multiple bacteremia (which occurs in 5-10% of cases) may be delayed if the microscopic morphology of the two (or more) infecting strains is similar.

3. Normal bactericidal factors and antimicrobial agents in blood may continue to act in the culture and thus prevent or delay growth.

4. Certain fastidious organisms such as anaerobes or cell-wall deficient forms may not grow in conventional media.

Problem-Oriented Approach to Blood Culturing

There are several problems which must be taken into consideration for optimum results with blood cultures:

1. *Low-level bacteremia.* Table 3-I presents data from a study reported by Finegold *et al.* (1). Note that over half of

36

TABLE 3-I

COLONY COUNTS IN WHOLE BLOOD POUR PLATES

Type of organism	No. of positive cultures	Median colony count/ml whole blood	No. of cultures with very low counts	
			No. with counts of 1 or less per ml	No. with counts of 1-10/ml
Gram-positive	25	·8	8 (6)[a]	5 (1)[a]
Gram-negative	25	1	13 (9)	9 (9)
Fungus	4	18	2 (0)	0
Total	54	7	23 (15)	14 (10)

a: number on antimicrobial therapy at time of culture indicated in parentheses.

positive cultures with gram-negative bacilli (all clinically significant bacteremias) had colony counts of only 1 organism or less per ml of whole blood. Antimicrobial therapy was being used in most of these patients; however, the problem is a real one as the patients in this study were unselected except as they were likely candidates for a positive blood culture. The best solution to this problem would seem to be to draw as much blood as possible for culture. However, there are limitations to this approach. In the broth and pour plate techniques, the blood must be diluted significantly by the medium (see below); therefore, one would need to set up several broths or many pour plates.

2. *Bactericidal power of blood.* Normal serum factors kill bacteria within seconds (2), so that unless this effect is diluted out or neutralized *immediately,* growth of any bacteria present in a blood sample may be prevented or delayed. Since 10 percent serum also kills bacteria, though more slowly (40 minutes), it is apparent that the usual 1:10 dilution of blood in broth culture media is not adequate. One must dilute to at least 1:20, and preferably more, to counteract this effect.

Another approach to this problem is neutralization of the

Bacteremia

TABLE 3-II

EFFECT OF SODIUM POLYANETHOL SULFONATE (SPS) ON RECOVERY
OF BACTERIA FROM BROTH BLOOD CULTURES°

	With SPS	Without SPS
Positive	17	12
Faster growth	2	0
More luxuriant growth	6	0

° 100 blood cultures. Albimi Brucella broth was used.

bactericidal activity. Citrate is effective in this regard but is, itself, toxic for many gram-positive organisms (3). Heparin is effective, without toxicity, but sodium polyanethol sulfonate (Liquoid) is preferable because it withstands autoclaving. Polyanethol sulfonate was first noted to possess this activity in 1938 and has been used in blood cultures in Great Britain for many years. However, controlled trials in clinical blood culture studies were not performed until recently (3, 4). These studies show convincingly that this substance significantly increases yields in clinical blood culture work. This is illustrated in Table 3-II, adapted from Finegold *et al.* (4). Polyanethol sulfonate is of no value in pour plate cultures. This substance is inhibitory to some strains of anaerobic streptococci, *H. influenzae,* gonococci, meningococci, and viridans streptococci. Unpublished data from our laboratory (Attebery and Finegold) showed complete inhibition of 2 and partial inhibition of 4 of 15 anaerobic or microaerophilic cocci or streptococci by 0.03-0.05% polyanethol sulfonate.

Still another way to counteract the bactericidal power of blood is to use a membrane filter blood culture system (5) which physically removes bacteria from the blood and, therefore, from inhibitory substances therein. Our initial studies of this technique (1, 5) showed enhanced speed of recovery (in comparison with broth and pour plate cultures) despite a cumbersome technique (involving sedimentation of red blood cells and filtration of plasma and white blood cells) which permitted use of only 3 ml of blood as a rule. These studies encompassed 277 clinical blood cultures, 70 of which were positive by one or more techniques. The filters were positive in an average of 28 hours, compared to 46 hours for the pour plate and 61 hours for the broth cultures. In the case of the broth cultures, additional time was required, of course, for growth of subcultures on solid media. With this early, crude technique, the total number of positive cultures was lower with the filter technique than with the other two procedures. Another advantage of the filter technique, aside from speed of recovery of organisms (in the form of colonies with typical morphology), was the availability of colonial growth for rapid bacteriologic and biochemical tests which permitted probable identification within two hours in most cases (5).

Subsequently, others have introduced modifications of the membrane filter procedure utilizing dilution and filtration (6) and lysis of whole blood followed by filtration (7). Unpublished data from our laboratory reveals very significant loss of bacteria with these two modifications. We have also modified our own procedure, originally by the use of filters with a larger diameter and larger pore sizes, and more recently with a lysed whole blood process which permits total recovery of bacteria present. This latter procedure, details of which will be published elsewhere, permits the use of 10 ml of blood and complete processing takes only 5 minutes or less. This practical system for membrane filtration will be available commercially in the form of a simple, disposable kit from McGaw Laboratories. The new lysed blood membrane filtration system was evaluated in patients undergoing genitourinary tract manipulation and was roughly comparable to conventional broth and pour plate systems in terms of total numbers of positives recovered while exhibiting faster growth more frequently (8). A more recent study, with further improvements in technique, involved hospitalized patients with suspected bacteremia (9). Among 94 patients, 18 had a positive blood culture by one technique or another. The filter was positive in 14 cases, 5 of which provided the fastest recovery (average of over 24 hours sooner than by the next fastest procedure). Furthermore, 7 of the 14 cultures were positive only on the filter. The next best techniques yielded 8 positives each. This study is continuing in order to expand the limited data available on clinical evaluation.

3. *Antimicrobial drugs in blood.* The problem presented here is similar to the one just discussed (normal bactericidal

power of blood). Evidence cited earlier (1) indicates that a significant percentage of patients on whom blood cultures are drawn are on antimicrobial drugs. It is not uncommon for such agents to prevent or delay growth of bacteria in blood cultures while failing to control the responsible infection (particularly when other therapy such as surgical drainage is required). Again, the solutions to the problem are dilution (preferably at least 1:20 or 1:30), inactivation, or removal of organisms from the blood by membrane filtration. Inactivation is not always possible, but certain agents may be eliminated in this way. Paraamino- benzoic acid effectively neutralizes sulfonamides, while penicil- linase neutralizes penicillin. Large amounts of penicillinase are required in the case of penicillinase-resistant penicillins and cephalosporins. Polymyxin, and aminoglycosides such as strep- tomycin, kanamycin and gentamicin are antagonized by poly- anethol sulfonate (10, 11); the antagonism varies from one type of medium to another in the case of the aminoglycosides and is most impressive in nutrient broth. The membrane filtration procedure, of course, removes bacteria from the inhibitory agents in the blood, although washing of the filter is necessary with the sedimentation-filtration system (see Figure 3-1).

4. *Clotting of blood.* Although clot culture has been used for recovery of *S. typhi,* blood specimens which clot generally give poor results in blood culture work. The organisms may either not be recovered or the time required to recover them may be greatly increased. Certain anticoagulants, such as ammonium oxalate or sodium citrate, are unsatisfactory because they are inhibitory to bacteria. Heparin and sodium polyanethol sulfonate are effective anticoagulants and the latter, in particular, is a good choice for other reasons previously discussed.

5. *Problem of contaminants.* Such common contaminants of blood cultures as *Staphylococcus epidermidis, Micrococcus* and diphtheroids are also capable of causing endocarditis in patients with damaged heart valves and of causing sustained bacteremia in patients with implanted prostheses (such as ventriculoatrial shunts). Quantitation of bacteremia by membrane filter or pour plate technique may allow distinction between contaminants and infecting organisms (several colonies/ml of blood would likely

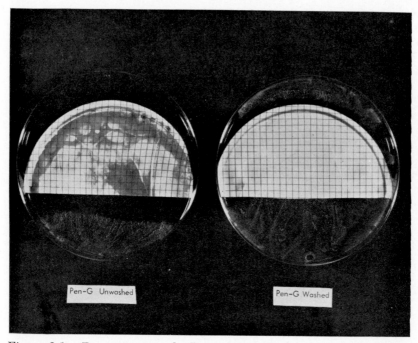

Figure 3-1. Demonstration of effectiveness of washing filter in removal of inhibitory substance (using sedimentation-plasma filtration procedure). Penicillin is added to blood sample in final concentration of 1 unit/ml. Plasma is filtered through two filters (following red cell sedimentation), one of which is subsequently washed. Halves of each filter are placed on blood agar plates surface-streaked with penicillin-sensitive organism. Filter at left is very inhibitory to test organism (residual penicillin), while filter at right shows only slight zone of inhibition at upper edge (which cannot be washed effectively because of O-ring).

mean true infection); however, more data is needed on levels of bacteremia in these types of infection. Presence of the same species or type of organism repeatedly in a sequence of blood cultures drawn separately, and preferably over an interval of several days, would speak for infection. Use of careful skin cleansing technique and aseptic technique throughout the culture procedure is very important. Finally, the clinical features must be taken into consideration in making a final decision.

6. *Need for rapid recovery and identification of organisms.* Typically, patients with bacteremia are among the sickest of

patients. Prompt diagnosis of the infection and identification of the organism(s) involved (and perhaps determination of the organism's susceptibility to various antimicrobial agents) greatly increase chances of effecting a cure and avoiding such complications of sepsis as shock, disseminated intravascular coagulation and metastatic infection. The importance of the membrane filter procedure in early detection and identification of organisms in bacteremia has already been stressed in item 2 above.

7. *Multiple bacteremia.* Simultaneous bacteremia with two or more organisms is not a rare phenomenon; it is seen in 5 to 10 percent of all bacteremias. Multiple bacteremia is more common in patients with malignancy or other debilitating disease and in patients who have undergone extensive surgery. Such patients, of course, exhibit a high mortality with bacteremia so that early, appropriate therapy becomes extremely important. As indicated earlier, the membrane filter blood culture (and pour plate culture, to a lesser extent) is particularly useful in detecting this type of bacteremia early. In broth cultures, if two different gram-negative bacilli were present this would usually not be apparent until after subculture (to solid media) of the positive broth; this would mean an unnecessary delay of 12 to 24 hours in addition to the slower growth initially in broth as compared to filters.

8. *Need for special techniques for certain organisms.* Among the organisms with special growth requirements which may be found in bacteremia, anaerobes are by far the most common. Marcoux *et al.* (12) isolated *Bacteroides* from 40 blood cultures in a 10 month period at the Mayo Clinic. Pankey (13) indicated that *Bacteroides* was the second commonest isolate from blood cultures at the Ochsner Clinic. Most of the commercially available broths advertised as anaerobic are not truly anaerobic (usually, 10 percent of the atmosphere has been replaced by carbon dioxide). Attebery and Finegold (14) described a pre-reduced broth bottled with a self-contained anaerobic atmosphere which is effective for growing anaerobes. This broth, when osmotically stabilized with sucrose and magnesium sulfate, is excellent for both anaerobes and cell-wall-deficient bacteria (L

forms). It is our present feeling that any good broth which is bottled by the pre-reduced anaerobically sterilized (PRAS) technique and which is osmotically stabilized is satisfactory.

In patients undergoing urinary tract manipulation (9) this PRAS osmotically stabilized broth (which also incorporated polyanethol sulfonate) picked up 8 anaerobic bacteria and two protoplasts not recovered in other broth media, pour plates, or on a membrane filter. Surprisingly, this broth also picked up significantly more conventional bacteria than all other systems. This might mean that these latter organisms orginally had minor cell-wall deficiencies no longer apparent after isolation or that sucrose and/or magnesium sulfate was useful as a growth factor. However, Muschel and Larsen (18) have shown that hypertonic sucrose is anticomplementary and this may explain its effect.

The advantage of the osmotically stabilized anaerobic broth was not apparent in the early results of our latest clinical study (8) in which, as previously indicated, the filter system was distinctly better, both in terms of total positive cultures and in speed of recovery. This lack of effect of the hypertonic anaerobic broth was at least partially explained by the fact that a number of the isolates in this recent study were obligate aerobes.

Other organisms, rarely encountered, with special growth requirements (viz., *Leptospira*) will have to be dealt with individually, when suspected clinically.

Ideal Blood Culture System

The combination of the filter technique and the anaerobic osmotically stabilized broth (without polyanethol sulfonate) makes an ideal system for blood cultures.

Ten ml of blood is drawn directly into a tube containing polyanethol sulfonate (final concentration of 0.05%) for the filter process. It is then placed into the special lysing solution which promptly effects total lysis. The entire solution is then filtered through a special apparatus with three individual membrane filters. One filter is placed on the surface of a blood agar plate and another on chocolate agar, both to be incubated under 10 percent CO_2. The third filter is placed on eosin methylene blue (or similar) medium and is incubated aerobically.

The advantages of the membrane filter blood culture technique are:

1. Much more rapid growth
2. Initial growth is in the form of characteristic colonies (saving a subculture step and therefore an additional 12-24 hours)
3. Differential and selective media may be used directly
4. Colonies on filter may be used directly for rapid identification and susceptibility studies
5. Inhibitory substances in blood (normal antibacterial factors and antimicrobial drugs) may be eliminated
6. Quantitation of bacteremia
7. Early recognition of multiple bacteremia
8. Ultimately, techniques may be developed (viz., fluorescent antibody procedures) to permit direct recognition or even identification of organisms trapped in the filter, without prior incubation

The anaerobic osmotically stabilized broth was designed primarily to recover anaerobes and protoplasts but, as indicated, grows conventional bacteria well also. Even certain obligate aerobes, such as *Pseudomonas aeruginosa,* will grow well in it because of the presence of potassium nitrate which can be metabolized anaerobically. Five ml of blood can be put promptly into 95 ml of this broth or 10 ml of blood can be used with 190 ml of medium (1:20 dilution of blood).

The two setups (filter and broth) complement each other well and provide a complete system; pour plates are not needed. Other specialized systems would be necessary only when an unusual pathogen, with very special growth requirements, may be suspected on clinical or epidemiological grounds.

Other Techniques for Rapid Detection of Bacteremia

Several other cultural and non-cultural techniques for detection (and identification, also, in some cases) of bacteremia have been proposed. The potential speed of these procedures (because of elimination of, or reduction in, time needed for incubation) would represent a big advantage over cultural procedures.

One of these newer procedures is early detection of bacterial growth in broth containing C^{14}-labeled glucose by means of monitoring for liberated $^{14}CO_2$ (15). This procedure, of course,

offers no clue as to the identity of the organism. Another evaluation of the radiometric detection system (16) failed to confirm the
earlier claims made for it; this latter study included both artificially seeded blood (various inocula up to 4,250 organisms/ml)
and a limited clinical trial. However, this radiometric system
has been changed in several ways (different media composition
and introduction of a CO_2 *wash* of the bottles) subsequently.

Another promising procedure is the use of gas chromatography
to detect metabolites resulting from bacterial growth (17). This
procedure could, theoretically, yield positive results without
incubation or at least after short incubation periods. It might
also provide specific identification of organisms on the basis of
characteristic patterns of volatile end-products of metabolism.
Unfortunately, here too, one attempt to utilize this approach
with clinical blood cultures failed to demonstrate any benefit
from the chromatographic procedure (8). End-products of
bacterial metabolism such as volatile fatty acids and acetoin
were detected in some positive blood cultures, but never prior to
the time that the cultures were noted to be positive by gross
inspection. An electron capture detector was used in addition to
flame ionization and thermal conductivity detectors. Perhaps
the use of other media or other column packings might have
led to better results.

REFERENCES

1. Finegold, S. M.; White, M. L.; Ziment, I., and Winn, W. R.: Rapid
   diagnosis of bacteremia. *Appl Microbiol, 18*:458, 1969.
2. Lowrance, B. L., and Traub, W. H.: Inactivation of the bactericidal
   activity of human serum by Liquoid (sodium polyanetholsulfonate).
   Appl Microbiol, 17:839, 1969.
3. Rosner, R.: Effect of various anticoagulants and no anticoagulant on
   ability to isolate bacteria directly from parallel clinical blood
   specimens. *Am J Clin Path, 49*:216, 1968.
4. Finegold, S. M.; Ziment, I.; White, M. L.; Winn, W. R., and Carter,
   W. T.: Evaluation of polyanethol sulfonate (Liquoid) in blood
   cultures. In *Antimicrobial Agents and Chemotherapy—1967* (Hobby,
   G. L., ed.). American Society for Microbiology, p. 692, 1968.
5. Winn, W. R.; White, M. L.; Carter, W. T.; Miller, A. B., and Finegold,
   S. M.: Rapid diagnosis of bacteremia with quantitative differential-
   membrane filtration culture. *JAMA, 197*:539, 1966.

6. Kozub, W. R.; Kirkham, W. R.; Chatman, C. E., and Pribor, H. C.: A practical blood culturing method employing dilution and filtration. *Am J Clin Path,* 52:105, 1969.
7. Rose, R. E., and Bradley, W. J.: Using the membrane filter in clinical microbiology. *Medical Lab,* 3:22, 1969.
8. Sullivan, N. M.; Sutter, V. L.; Attebery, H. R., and Finegold, S. M.: Clinical evaluation of improved blood culture procedures. Abstr. Annual Meet., Am. Soc. Microbiol. 1972, p. 87.
9. Sullivan, N. M.; Sutter, V. L.; Carter, W. T.; Attebery, H. R., and Finegold, S. M.: Bacteremia after genito-urinary tract manipulation. I. Bacteriologic aspects and evaluation of various blood culture systems. *Appl Microbiol.* 23:1101, 1972.
10. Traub, W. H.: Antagonism of polymyxin B and kanamycin sulfate by Liquoid (sodium polyanetholsulfonate) *in vitro. Experientia,* 25:206, 1969.
11. Traub, W. H., and Lowrance, B. L.: Media-dependent antagonism of gentamicin sulfate by Liquoid (sodium polyanetholsulfonate). *Experientia,* 25:1184, 1969.
12. Marcoux, J. A.; Zabransky, R. J.; Washington, J. A., II; Wellman, W. E., and Martin, W. J.: Bacteroides bacteremia. *Minn Med,* 53:1169, 1970.
13. Pankey, G. A.: Personal communication, 1971.
14. Attebery, H. R., and Finegold, S. M.: A new anaerobic blood culture system. *Proc X International Congress for Microbiology,* Mexico City, 105, 1970.
15. De Land, F. H., and Wagner, H. N., Jr.: Early detection of bacterial growth, with carbon-14-labeled glucose. *Radiology,* 92:154, 1969.
16. Washington, J. A., II, and Yu, P. K. W.: Radiometric method for detection of bacteremia. *Appl Microbiol,* 22:100, 1971.
17. Mitruka, B. M., and Alexander, M.: Rapid and sensitive detection of bacteria by gas chromatography. *Appl Microbiol,* 16:636, 1968.
18. Muschel, L. H., and Larsen, L. J.: Effect of hypertonic sucrose upon the immune bactericidal reaction. *Infection and Immunity,* 1:51, 1970.

CHAPTER 4

BACTEREMIA DUE TO ANAEROBIC, UNUSUAL AND FASTIDIOUS BACTERIA

JOHN A. WASHINGTON II, M.D.

Anaerobic Bacteria

THE FREQUENCY AND therapeutic implications of bacteremias due to anaerobic bacteria have been increasingly recognized in recent years (1, 2, 3, 4, 5, 6). In a review, concluded in December 1970, of the distribution of organisms responsible for bacteremia at the Mayo Clinic and affiliated hospitals during a 2½-year evaluation of two different blood culture media, anaerobic bacteria represented 13 percent of positive cultures, excluding presumed contaminants, and 20 percent of patients with bacteremia (7). Members of the family Bacteroidaceae constituted 78 percent of the cultures with anaerobic bacteria and 69 percent of the patients with anaerobic bacteremias. The Bacteroidaceae were not speciated until 1970; however, in 1970, 77 percent of the isolates in this family were identified as *B. fragilis*.

Data on 123 patients at this institution with bacteremias due to the Bacteroidaceae have been reported recently (4). During the 10-year period March 1959 through June 1969, these 123 patients had a total of 285 positive cultures. In 23.6 percent of the patients at least one other organism was isolated from the blood concurrently, and in 29.2 percent, Bacteroidaceae were isolated from specimens from other sites. Fifty-nine percent of the patients were seen in the first 8 years of the study and 41 percent in the last 2 years.

Prior to the middle of 1968 a dextrose-brain broth (DBB) and pour plates were utilized for routine blood cultures. In

47

1968, use of Thiol and Tryptic Soy (TSB) Broths (Difco) under vacuum with added CO_2 was begun; blood was inoculated into these media on a 10 percent (w/v) basis. For 2 months, Thiol and TSB were evaluated in parallel with DBB. Of the eight specimens from which Bacteroidaceae were isolated, Thiol was positive for all eight, TSB for five, and DBB for one. In the one instance in which all three media were positive, Thiol and TSB became positive within 48 hours and DBB became positive in 10 days. On a more extensive evaluation of relative isolation rates in Thiol and TSB between 1968 and 1970, there was no statistically significant difference between the two media (Table 4-I). Mean times for detection of positivity were 3.8 days in TSB and 4.2 days in Thiol. More recent data from our laboratory comparing TSB and Thioglycollate-135C (BBL) are shown in Table 4-II.

Of the 123 patients studied by Marcoux and co-workers (4), 66.6 percent were in their fifth, sixth, or seventh decade of life. Most (62%) had underlying gastrointestinal conditions, and, of this group, most had colonic malignancies. Other underlying colonic conditions included diverticulitis, polyps, and chronic ulcerative colitis. Small bowel and gastric problems included malignancy, obstruction, perforation, ulceration, and fistulae. Eighteen percent of the patients had underlying genitourinary problems, of which half represented malignancies. Finally, 20

TABLE 4-I

COMPARISON OF ISOLATION RATES OF BACTEROIDACEAE FROM
THIOL AND TRYPTICASE SOY (TSB) BROTHS, 1968 TO 1970

Result in	Result in TSB		
Thiol	Pos.	Neg.	Total
Pos.	182	76	258
Neg.	74	0	74
Total	256	76	332

TABLE 4-II

COMPARISON OF ISOLATION RATES OF BACTEROIDACEAE FROM
TRYPTICASE SOY (TSB) AND THIOGLYCOLLATE-135C
BROTHS, JANUARY TO JUNE 1971

Result in Thioglycollate	Result in TSB		Total
	Pos.	Neg.	
Pos.	32	11	43
Neg.	13	0	13
Total	45	11	56

percent had miscellaneous conditions consisting of diseases of
the skin or subcutaneous tissues or of the cardiovascular, central
nervous, hematopoietic, skeletal, or connective tissue system.
Precipitating factors of the bacteremias in 101 patients included
antecedent diagnostic or surgical procedures, mainly of the
gastrointestinal tract.

The signs and symptoms of bacteremia, which were similar
to those encountered with other gram-negative bacillary bacteremias, ensued within 1 week of a procedure in 50 percent
of the patients. Overall mortality was 28.5 percent. In a group
of 49 patients who received antibiotics with surgical drainage,
14 percent of the tetracycline-treated and 9 percent of the
chloramphenicol-treated patients died. In a group of 39 patients
treated with antibiotics alone, 35 percent of the tetracycline-
treated and 80 percent of the chloramphenicol-treated patients
died. More recent analysis of such data suggests that those not
treated surgically represented a sicker group of patients, frequently in shock and with oliguria or anuria. In a group of 19
patients treated by incision and drainage only, approximately
84 percent survived. Finally, in a group of 16 patients who
received neither surgical nor antibiotic therapy, 50 percent died.
The choice of treatment and its outcome obviously were influenced by the severity of the illness.

Other anaerobic bacteria frequently encountered in blood cultures include *Propionibacterium acnes* which is rarely of any clinical significance and probably represents a skin contaminant. In a 2½-year experience with blood cultures reported by Washington (7), clostridia were isolated in 44 instances from 30 patients, anaerobic streptococci (*Peptostreptococcus*) were isolated in 27 instances from 16 patients, and members of the genus *Peptococcus* were isolated in 13 instances from 12 patients. *Veillonella, Bifidobacterium eriksonii,* and *Eubacterium lentum* were isolated from one, four, and two patients, respectively.

Alpern and Dowell (5) described an association between *Clostridium septicum* infection and the presence of an underlying malignancy in 23 of 27 patients from whom this organism had been recovered. In 21 of these patients, *C. septicum* was isolated from the blood. Prompt antimicrobial therapy appeared to be highly effective in preventing death. The same authors (8) reviewed the clinical histories of 86 patients with non-histotoxic clostridial bacteremia, the most common etiologic agents of which were *Clostridium* NCDC group P-1, *C. tertium, C. paraputrificum, C. bifermentans, C. subterminale, C. multifermentans* and *C. sordellii.* Bacteremias due to these clostridial species were commonly associated with intra-abdominal lesions, diseases of the hematologic, genitourinary, and cardiac systems, a history of recent surgery or intercurrent antibiotic therapy, and malignancies. The clinical picture resembled that of gram-negative sepsis and did not appear to be favorably affected by antimicrobial therapy.

It is important, therefore, for both the clinician and the laboratorian to be aware of the facts that an appreciable number of bacteremias are due to anaerobes, that the usual antibiotic treatment with a penicillin or cephalosporin and an aminoglycoside would not be effective against anaerobic gram-negative bacilli on the basis of *in vitro* susceptibility data (9) and that, in nearly 25 percent of instances of bacteremia due to anaerobic gram-negative bacilli, other bacteria will be present (4).

Polymicrobial bacteremia is another problem of which both the clinician and the laboratorian must be aware. According to Hermans and Washington (10) and Washington (7) it occurs in at least 6 percent of patients with bacteremia. Obviously, the possibilities of occurrence of polymicrobial bacteremia or of bacteremia due to anaerobes in pure or mixed culture present quite a challenge.

Felner and Dowell (11) recently reported clinical and bacteriologic data from 33 cases of endocarditis due to anaerobic bacteria. Species of *Bacteroides* and *Fusobacterium* accounted for 18 of the 33 cases. There were five cases of endocarditis due to *P. acnes,* each substantiated by a minimum of two positive blood cultures.

Unusual and Fastidious Bacteria

Endocarditis provides a useful point of departure from anaerobic bacteremias to bacteremias due to organisms with special growth requirements or to unusual bacteria. Facklam and Moody (12) of the Center for Disease Control studied 84 strains of *Streptococcus mutans,* 11 of which were isolated from blood. Four of these were from patients at the Mayo institutions with subacute bacterial endocarditis. Since then we have isolated *S. mutans* from the blood of six additional patients. The major criteria for recognizing *S. mutans* are the production of acid from mannitol and typical distinguishing colonies on 5 percent sucrose agar. These organisms give a positive bile-esculin reaction but fail to precipitate in Lancefield group D extract. The organism is a constituent of the normal flora of the mouth and has been isolated from the blood of patients with a history of dental procedures (13, 14).

Page and King (15) reported 23 and 15 cases, respectively, of endocarditis due to *Actinobacillus actinomycetemcomitans* and *Haemophilus aphrophilus.* In our own recent experience, we have encountered three cases of endocarditis due to the former and two of endocarditis due to the latter. Sutter and Finegold (16) recently described the growth factor and atmospheric requirements of these organisms, as well as of *Bacteroides corrodens* (HB-1) which we have isolated from blood in rare instances. These organisms grow poorly aerobically and appear to grow better under anaerobic conditions with added CO_2. *H. aphrophilus* does not require hemin (X factor) or diphosphopyridine nucleotide (V factor) for growth. Since *B corrodens* has been found to be a facultative anaerobe (17, 18) its taxonomic status has been questioned and remains uncertain.

Cardiobacterium hominis (IId) can be readily confused with *A. actinomycetemcomitans* and *H. aphrophilus.* It has caused endocarditis (19, 20, 21). The differentiating biochemical reactions of these three organisms are listed in Table 4-III. *A. actinomycetemcomitans* and *H. aphrophilus* may be readily differentiated from each other by means of the catalase test and fermentation of lactose and from *C. hominis* by the cytochrome oxidase and indole tests. These bacteria have been isolated from a variety of liquid blood culture media but especially from thioglycollate.

Another unusual organism which we have isolated from the blood of a patient with fatal endocarditis is *Vibrio fetus* (22). Bokkenheuser (23) reviewed the European and American literature since 1947 and found 64 reported cases of *V. fetus* infection, to which he added 10 new cases. In 91 percent of

TABLE 4-III

BIOCHEMICAL CHARACTERISTICS OF *Actinobacillus actinomycetemcomitans,* *Haemophilus aphrophilus,* AND *Cardiobacterium hominis*

Test	A. actinomycetemcomitans	H. aphrophilus	C. hominis
Catalase	+	−	−
Cytochrome oxidase	−	−	+
NO$_3$ reduction	+	+	−
Indole	−	−	+
Acid produced from			
Lactose	−	+·	−
Sucrose	−	+	+
Xylose	+(−)	−	−
Mannitol	+(−)	−	+(−)
Sorbitol	−	−	+

the 74 cases the organism was recovered from blood. Morphologically, *V. fetus* is a small, short, curved, gram-negative rod with a tendency to filament formation on repeated subculture. It is fastidious in its growth requirements and is strictly microaerophilic when first isolated. It generally fails to grow on blood agar plates in the absence of CO_2. *V. fetus* is fairly inactive biochemically (Table 4-IV) but generally does give positive cytochrome oxidase, catalase, nitrate reductase, and motility tests. King (24) described a group of organisms resembling *Vibrio* but serologically distinct from *V. fetus* and referred to as *related vibrios*. They are differentiated from *V. fetus* by their inability to grow at 25 C and their ability to grow at 42 C.

The annual reported incidence of brucellosis has been progressively diminishing in the last decade (Annual Supplement, Morbidity and Mortality, Center for Disease Control, U.S. Department of Health, Education and Welfare, Summary 1970). It appears that as the incidence of this disease decreases its diagnosis becomes more difficult. In its bacteremic form at this institution, *B. abortus* has been the most common species isolated, with *B. suis* accounting for most localized lesions. Golden *et al.*

TABLE 4-IV

BIOCHEMICAL REACTIONS OF *Vibrio fetus*

Test	Result	Test	Result
Cytochrome oxidase	+	Growth at 25 C	+
Catalase	+	Growth at 42 C	–
NO_3 reduction	+	Carbohydrate fermentation	–
MR/VP	–/–	Carbohydrate oxidation	–
Citrate	–		
Urea	–	Gelatin liquefaction	–
		Motility	+

described in 1970 (25) a case of *B. suis* endocarditis which is important because there has been only one previous case of endocarditis reported as being due to this species. Recently, a farmer in perfect health came to the Mayo Clinic for a "brucella checkup" because his cattle had been aborting. A single blood culture drawn to comply with his wishes grew out *B. abortus.* This infectious disease may be dying out, but it certainly is not dead yet.

Blood cultures for brucella may be performed several ways. One is to add 5 to 10 ml of blood to about 75 ml of Albimi, tryptose, or trypticase soy broth in a cotton-stoppered flask, incubate in an atmosphere of 10 percent CO_2, and subculture at regular intervals to solid media, such as trypticase soy agar, which are incubated in an atmosphere of 10 percent CO_2 for up to 6 weeks. Alternatively, one may use Castañeda double medium which may be prepared easily as described by Sonnenwirth (26) or purchased commercially. Basically, this medium consists of a bottle containing an agar slant and a liquid medium. The bottle may be stoppered and its dead space adjusted to contain 10 percent CO_2. Instead of subculturing the broth to agar, one simply tips this bottle two or three times a week so that the broth flows over the agar.

There are a number of bacteria which have been infrequently reported as causes of bacteremia but which do not necessarily have special growth requirements. Identification of these organisms usually is contingent upon the use of an adequate number of appropriate biochemical tests.

The isolation of *Yersinia enterocolitica* from blood has been reported recently by Sonnenwirth (27), Chessum *et al.* (28) and Mollaret *et al.* (29). This organism may be readily confused with certain genera of the family Enterobacteriaceae. The triple sugar-iron agar (TSIA) reaction is usually acidic on the slant (due to sucrose fermentation) and acidic in the butt (due to glucose fermentation). Occasional strains, however, may yield an alkaline/acidic TSIA reaction since not all biotypes ferment sucrose (30). Hydrogen sulfide (H_2S) is not produced in TSIA. Other biochemical reactions are listed in Table 4-V.

TABLE 4-V

BIOCHEMICAL CHARACTERISTICS OF *Yersinia enterocolitica**

Test	Result	Test	Result
Simmons' citrate	−	Nitrate reduction	+
Christensen's urea	+	Indole	d†
Lysine decarboxylase	−	β−Galactosidase (ONPG)	d
Arginine dihydrolase	−	Fermentation	
Ornithine decarboxylase	+	Glucose	+
Phenylalanine deaminase	−	Sucrose	+
Malonate utilization	−	Mannitol	+
Oxidase	−	Maltose	+
Catalase	+	Arabinose	+
Methyl red	+	Sorbitol	+
Voges-Proskauer		Lactose	−
25 C	+	Adonitol	−
37 C	−	Dulcitol	−
Motility		Raffinose	−
25 C	+	Rhamnose	−
37 C			

* Adapted from Niléhn (30).
† d = different biochemical reactions.

Septicemia due to *Edwardsiella tarda* has been reported by Jordan and Hadley (31) and by Sonnenwirth (27). This organism, which belongs in the family Enterobacteriaceae, yields an alkaline/acidic reaction and produces H_2S in TSIA. It possesses lysine and ornithine decarboxylases but not arginine dihydrolase, phenylalanine deaminase, or urease. It produces indole and is methyl red-positive but Voges-Proskauer-negative. It does not utilize citrate or acetate as its sole source of carbon. It ferments glucose but not mannitol.

Members of the genus *Erwinia*, more specifically those

grouped under Herbicola-lathyri, have attracted considerable
attention recently as etiologic agents in nosocomially acquired
bacteremias as reported by von Graevenitz (32, 33) and in
Morbidity and Mortality, Center for Disease Control, U.S.
Department of Health, Education and Welfare, Mar. 20, 1971.
No such strains have been isolated from blood at this institution,
but they are commonly isolated from cultures of wounds incurred
in farming accidents. Ewing and Edwards (34) have indicated
that *Erwinia,* as presented in Bergey's Manual (35), is composed
of four groups: (1) the true *Erwinia (E. amylovora* and related
species) which should be classified in the tribe Erwineae and
the family Erwiniaceae; (2) the pectolytic bacteria (formerly
E. carotovorum) which should be placed in the genus *Pecto-
bacterium* of the family Klebsielleae; (3) a heterogeneous collection of microorganisms identifiable as *Enterobacter* or *Klebsiella;*
and (4) a group of microorganisms composed of the Herbicola-
lathyri bacteria. It is this last group of *Erwinia* which Ewing
and Fife (36) think resemble members of the genus *Enterobacter*
sufficiently to warrant the proposal that they be incorporated
into this genus as an additional species, *E. agglomerans.* Most of
these organisms produce a yellow pigment, and all are fermenta-
tive. A selected list of biochemical reactions of this group of
organisms is presented in Table 4-VI. In our own experience
(Pien *et al.,* unpublished observations, 1971), nearly 75 percent
of these organisms have been anaerogenic; in the anaerogenic
group, slightly over 50 percent have produced an alkaline/acidic
TSIA reaction.

In tropical or subtropical regions, sepsis with hepatic abscess
formation has appeared to be characteristic of most fatal cases
of *Chromobacterium violaceum* (37). Additional such cases
have been reported by Ognibene and Thomas in 1970 (38) and
Johnson and co-workers in 1971 (39). This organism is a gram-
negative bacillus which grows on eosin-methylene blue agar and
MacConkey agar and which usualy produces a violet pigment.
Oxidase is usually present but may be weak or even absent. Other
positive biochemical reactions (Weaver, personal communication,
1970) include: catalase, citrate utilization, nitrate reduction,
gelatin liquefaction, milk peptonization, arginine dihydrolase,

TABLE 4-VI

SELECTED BIOCHEMICAL REACTIONS OF *Enterobacter agglomerans*
(Aerogenic and Anaerogenic Biogroups Combined)*

Test	Result†	Test	Result†
Simmons' citrate	d	Fermentation	
Christensen's urea	d	Glucose	+
Lysine decarboxylase	–	Lactose	d
Arginine dihydrolase	–	Sucrose	d
Ornithine decarboxylase	–	Dulcitol	d
Phenylalanine deaminase	– or +	Adonitol	–
Malonate utilization	+ or –	Inositol	d
Methyl red (37 C)	– or +	Sorbitol	d
Voges-Proskauer (37 C)	+ or –	Arabinose	+
KCN	– or +	Raffinose	d
Sodium pectate	–	Rhamnose	d
Nitrate reduction	+ or –	Maltose	+ or (+)
Oxidase	–		

* Adapted from Ewing and Fife (36) and unpublished observations of Pien *et al.* (1971).
† + = 90% or more positive within 48 hours' incubation; — = 90% or more negative within 48 hours' incubation; + or — = majority of strains positive; — or + = majority of strains negative; (+) = positive reaction after 3 or more days' incubation; d = different biochemical reactions.

motility, growth at 42 C, and fermentation of glucose, mannose, and trehalose. Most strains have produced an alkaline/acidic reaction in TSIA, but a few strains have produced an acidic/acidic reaction. A few strains have produced indole and have been methyl red-positive. *C. violaceum* may be confused with the Enterobacteriaceae, *Yersinia, Aeromonas,* and *Vibrio.*

CONCLUSION

A large number of diverse groups of unusual or fastidious bacteria may be isolated in cultures of blood. Their recognition is not only predicated upon the use of adequate cultural techniques but also upon the application and interpretation of appropriate biochemical tests. Because of these factors, their true frequency of occurrence is unknown. Only through an increasing awareness of the possibilities of their presence in bacteremias can adequate knowledge of their pathogenicity be obtained.

REFERENCES

1. Bornstein, D. L.; Weinberg, A. N., and Swartz, M. N., *et al.*: Anaerobic infections—review of current experience. *Medicine, 43*:207, 1964.
2. Bodner, S. J.; Koenig, M. G., and Goodman, J. S.: Bacteremic bacteroides infections. *Ann Intern Med, 73*:537, 1970.
3. Gelb, A. F., and Seligman, S. J.: Bacteroidaceae bacteremia: effect of age and focus of infection upon clinical course. *JAMA, 212*:1038, 1970.
4. Marcoux, J. A.; Zabransky, R. J.; Washington, J. A., II, *et al.*: Bacteroides bacteremia. *Minn Med, 53*:1169, 1970.
5. Alpern, R. J., and Dowell, V. R., Jr.: *Clostridium septicum* infections and malignancy. *JAMA, 209*:385, 1969.
6. Felner, J. M., and Dowell, V. R., Jr.: "Bactoerides" bacteremia. *Am J Med, 50*:787, 1971.
7. Washington, J. A., II: Comparison of two commercially available media for detection of bacteremia. *Appl Microbiol, 22*:604, 1971.
8. Alpern, R. J., and Dowell, V. R., Jr.: Nonhistotoxic clostridial bacteremia. *Am J Clin Pathol, 55*:717-722, 1971.
9. Martin, W. J.; Gardner, M., and Washington, J. A., II: *In vitro* antimicrobial susceptibility of anaerobic bacteria isolated from clinical specimens (abstract). Read at the 11th Interscience Conference on Antimicrobial Agents and Chemotherapy, Atlantic City, October 19 to 22, 1971.
10. Hermans, P. E., and Washington, J. A., II: Polymicrobial bacteremia. *Ann Intern Med, 73*:387, 1970.
11. Felner, J. M., and Dowell, V. R., Jr.: Anaerobic bacterial endocarditis. *N Engl J Med, 283*:1188, 1970.
12. Facklam, R. R., and Moody, M. D.: Report on *Streptococcus mutans* for members of the subcommittee on streptococci and pneumococci. Atlanta, Georgia, National Communicable Disease Center, June, 1970.
13. Edwardsson, S.: Characteristics of caries-inducing human streptococci resembling *Streptococcus mutans*. *Arch Oral Biol, 13*:637, 1968.
14. Carlsson, J.; Söderholm, G., and Almfeldt, I.: Prevalence of *Streptococcus sanguis* and *Streptococcus mutans* in the mouth of persons wearing full-dentures. *Arch Oral Biol, 14*:243, 1969.

15. Page, M. I., and King, E. O.: Infection due to *Actinobacillus actino-mycetemcomitans* and *Haemophilus aphrophilus*. *N Engl J Med,* 275:181, 1966.
16. Sutter, V. L., and Finegold, S. M.: *Haemophilus aphrophilus* infections: clinical and bacteriologic studies. *Ann NY Acad Sci, 174:468,* 1970.
17. Henriksen, S. D.: Corroding bacteria from the respiratory tract. 2. *Bacteroides corrodens. Acta Pathol Microbiol Scand,* 75:91, 1969.
18. Hill, L. R.; Snell, J. J. S., and Lapage, S. P.: Identification and characterisation of *Bacteroides corrodens. J Med Microbiol,* 3:483, 1970.
19. Slotnick, I. J., and Dougherty, M.: Further characterization of an unclassified group of bacteria causing endocarditis in man: *Cardiobacterium hominis. Antonie van Leeuwenhoek, 30:261,* 1964.
20. Snyder, A. I., and Ellner, P. D.: Cardiobacterium hominis endocarditis. *NY State J Med, 69:704,* 1969.
21. Midgley, J.; Lapage, S. P.; Jenkins, B. A. G., *et al.*: *Cardiobacterium hominis* endocarditis. *J Med Microbiol,* 3:91, 1970.
22. Lee, M. Y.; Ludwig, J., Geraci, J. E., *et al.*: Fatal *Vibrio fetus* endocarditis: report of one case and review of the literature. *Virchows Arch (Pathol Anat),* 350:87, 1970.
23. Bokkenheuser, V.: *Vibrio fetus* infection in man. I. Ten new cases and some epidemiologic observations. *Am J Epidemiol,* 91:400, 1970.
24. King, E. O.: The laboratory recognition of *Vibrio fetus* and a closely related *Vibrio* isolated from cases of human vibriosis. *Ann NY Acad Sci,* 98:700, 1962.
25. Golden, B.; Layman, T. E.; Koontz, F. P., *et al.*: *Brucella suis* endocarditis. *South Med J,* 63:392, 1970.
26. Sonnenwirth, A. C.: Media, tests and reagents. In *Gradwohl's Clinical Laboratory Methods and Diagnosis: A Textbook on Laboratory Procedures and Their Interpretation.* Vol. 2. Seventh edition. Edited by S. Frankel, S. Reitman, and A. C. Sonnenwirth. St. Louis, C. V. Mosby Company, 1970, pp. 1078-1121.
27. Sonnenwirth, A. C.: Bacteremia with and without meningitis due to *Yersinia enterocolitica, Edwardsiella tarda, Comamonas terrigena,* and *Pseudomonas maltophilia. Ann NY Acad Sci, 174:488,* 1970.
28. Chessum, B.; Frengley, J. D.; Fleck, D. G., *et al.*: Case of septicaemia due to Yersinia enterocolitica. *Br Med J,* 3:466, 1971.
29. Mollaret, H. H.; Omland, T.; Henriksen, S. D., *et al.*: Les septicémies humaines a Yersinia enterocolitica: a propos de dix sept cas récents. *Presse Med,* 79:345, 1971.
30. Niléhn, B.: Studies of *Yersinia enterocolitica* with special reference to bacterial diagnosis and occurrence in human acute enteric disease. *Acta Pathol Microbiol Scand* (Suppl), 206:5, 1969.
31. Jordan, G. W., and Hadley, W. K.: Human infection with *Edwardsiella tarda. Ann Intern Med,* 70:283, 1969.

32. von Graevenitz, A.: Part I. Gram-negative bacteria: *Erwinia* species isolates. *Ann NY Acad Sci, 174*:436, 1970.
33. von Graevenitz, A.: *Erwinia* infection from environmental sources (letter to the editor). *JAMA, 216*:1485, 1971.
34. Ewing, W. H., and Edwards, P. R.: *Identification of Enterobacteriaceae*. Third edition. Minneapolis, Burgess Publishing Co., 1972.
35. Breed, R. S.; Murray, E. G. D., and Smith, N. R.: *Bergey's Manual of Determinative Bacteriology*. Seventh edition. Baltimore, The Williams & Wilkins Company, 1957.
36. Ewing, W. H., and Fife, M. A.: *Enterobacter agglomerans*: the Herbicola-lathyri bacteria. Atlanta, Center for Disease Control, U.S. Department of Health, Education, and Welfare, 1971, pp. I-10, II-5.
37. Dauphinais, R. M., and Robben, G. G.: Fatal infection due to *Chromobacterium violaceum. Am J Clin Pathol, 50*:592, 1968.
38. Ognibene, A. J., and Thomas E.: Fatal infection due to *Chromobacterium violaceum* in Vietnam. *Am J Clin Pathol, 54*:607, 1970.
39. Johnson, W. M.; DiSalvo, A. F., and Steuer, R. R.: Fatal *Chromobacterium violaceum* septicemia. *Am J Clin Pathol, 56*:400, 1971.

CHAPTER 5

A QUANTITATIVE EVALUATION OF THREE DIFFERENT BLOOD CULTURE SYSTEMS

RICHARD ROSNER, M.S.

INTRODUCTION

THIS CHAPTER DEALS with the relationship between the physical condition of bacteria when present in the patient's bloodstream and the ability of the laboratory to recover such organisms from blood cultures. It also attempts to explore the possible interactions between the organisms, the patient's blood and the blood culture system.

In the past 40 years, much work has been published concerning the various clinical and microbiological aspects of bacteremia. Most of the microbiological literature has dealt with the problem of developing methods for early, rapid recovery of organisms from blood culture systems. Such areas as improvements of the base medium, new approaches to subculture methodology, the use of various atmospheres in blood culture systems, new methods for processing the specimen including membrane filtration, the use of multiple flask systems, and the employment of various additives in blood cultures have been explored but little has been reported about the physical condition of the bacterial organisms as they are introduced into various blood culture systems.

As early as 1925, Wright (1) discussed the then known facts and concepts of subacute infective endocarditis and its resulting bacteremia. Much of his report dealt with common problems, i.e., the timing and frequency of blood specimen collections, the significance of the organisms recovered, and methods for recovery of the organisms. Part of his report however, dealt with three

61

theoretical areas, namely: (1) The effect of normal inhibitory substances found in human blood on the ability to recover organisms, (2) the effect of phagocytes on bacteria in blood cultures, and (3) the reason for the often unpredictable delay in the lag phase of growth of some organisms in various blood culture systems. Wright concluded that the failure to recover organisms from blood cultures was often due to the continued action of phagocytes, and of inhibitory substances of the blood on the bacterial cells. He also stated that the delay in the growth of certain organisms in some blood cultures was due to a prolongation of their lag phase and that this prolongation was due to certain unknown peculiarities of the organisms which seemed to vary from species to species and from culture to culture. The studies described here were performed in order to attempt an explanation of these peculiarities and to demonstrate that the prolongation of the lag phase is due to the physical condition of the bacteria as they are placed into the blood culture system.

EXPERIMENTAL STUDIES

Methods

Three separate blood culture systems were employed. Each system utilized a single blood culture flask containing various medium/additive combinations. Each flask contained 45 ml of Brucella Broth (Pfizer). *Flask 1* contained the base medium, *Flask 2* contained the base medium plus Liquoid (Sodium poly-anethol sulfonate, Roche Diagnostics, Nutley, New Jersey), in a final concentration of 0.05%, and *Flask 3* contained the base medium, Liquoid, and sucrose in a final concentration of 30 percent.

The three flasks were inoculated by parallel culture technique. Since there were three separate flasks under study, for each blood culture requested, 15 ml of blood was drawn from the patient with a 20 ml syringe. Five ml aliquots of blood were placed into each of the three test flasks. This was done at the patient's bedside using skin preparation and inoculation methods previously described (2). Once inoculated, the three flasks were taped together and processed as a single unit. The flasks were incubated at 35° C for exactly four hours, at which time pour plates were prepared in duplicate from each flask in the unit. The pour plates were prepared by removing a 2 ml aliquot of the blood/medium mixture from each flask and placing one ml into each Petri dish. 24 ml of cooled Columbia Blood Agar base were then added to each dish. One set of pour plates were incubated for 48 hrs anaerobically and the other set for 24 hours in 4% CO_2. Total colony counts were obtained from all pour plates indicating growth. Immediately after preparing the pour plates, the sets of flasks were returned to the incubator and processed as previously described (2, 3). The process of preparing the pour plates at exactly four hours after collection of the specimen was carried out 24 hours a day and seven days a week in order to assure uniformity of methodology. The results obtained with cultures in which the pour plates were prepared either earlier or later than four hours were not included in this study.

Since the pour plates were prepared only four hours after collection of the specimen, it was assumed that those organisms which might be present would be in the lag phase of growth and therefore the number of colonies times 10 (blood/medium dilution factor) would represent the actual number of organisms present in the circulating blood of the patient at the time of collection. This assumption, as discussed below, was found to be invalid with regards to the gram negative enteric bacilli. In order to be included in this study, a patient had to have a minimum of three separate blood cultures with each of the flasks correctly inoculated. In order to be regarded as *positive*, at least one flask from each set of the patient's blood culture flasks had to yield growth, with the same species isolated from all of the patient's positive flasks.

Results

A total of 4,816 blood culture sets were obtained (14,448 individual blood culture flasks) during the study from 1,000 patients. A total of 261 patients were considered positive according to the criteria described. Of these, 140 patients yielded gram negative enteric bacilli and are not included in the results. From the remaining 121 patients' blood cultures, various gram positive and gram negative cocci, minute gram negative bacilli or anaerobic organisms were obtained. Table 5-I indicates the frequency with which each of the test flasks were found positive in the 121 patients.

TABLE 5-I

NUMBER OF PATIENTS WITH POSITIVE TEST MEDIA*

Flask I[a]	Flask II[b]	Flask III[c]
74	103	121

*: Total of 121 patients.
a: Base medium.
b: Base medium + sodium polyanethol sulfonate, 0.05%.
c: Base medium + sodium polyanethol sulfonate, 0.05% + sucrose, 30%.

Based on the quantitative results obtained from the pour plates, each positive patient was placed into one of three arbitrary groups. *Group 1* includes patients with less than 20 bacteria/ml of circulating blood, *Group 2* those with more than 20 but less than 100 organisms/ml of blood and *Group 3* those with more than 100 organisms/ml of blood. In those patients in whom more than one flask in a set was positive, the flask having the highest colony count was used to categorize the patient. Table 5-II indicates the number of patients falling into each of the arbitrary quantitative groups. Table 5-III indicates the number of patients found to be positive in each of the test media as determined by the quantitative results of the colony counts. The various organisms recovered and the number of patients found positive for each type of organism is shown in Table 5-IV. The frequency with which each organism was isolated is shown in Table 5-V, while Table 5-VI indicates the frequency of isolation for each organism from each of the three test media.

The gram negative enteric bacilli were excluded from the study because they were found to grow equally well in all three test systems, under the conditions employed here. No differences in the ability of either of the systems to allow recovery of these organisms were noted.

TABLE 5-II

NUMBER OF PATIENTS IN EACH QUANTITATIVE GROUP*

Group I[a]	Group II[b]	Group III[c]
22	39	60

*: Total of 121 patients.
a: < 20 organisms/ml blood.
b: 20-99 organisms/ml blood.
c: > 100 organisms/ml blood.

TABLE 5-III

NUMBER OF POSITIVE RECOVERIES FROM TEST MEDIA BASED ON
QUANTITATIVE RESULTS IN POUR PLATES

	Flask I[a]	Flask II[b]	Flask III[c]
Group I Patients (22)[d]	1	16	22
Group II Patients (39)[e]	22	31	39
Group III Patients (60)[f]	51	56	60

a: Base medium.
b: Base medium + sodium polyanethol sulfonate, 0.05%.
c: Base medium + sodium polyanethol sulfonate, 0.05% + sucrose, 30%.
d: < 20 organisms/ml blood.
e: 20-99 organisms/ml blood.
f: > 100 organisms/ml blood.

Discussion

According to the results obtained, if a single flask of Brucella Broth would have been used as the sole blood culture system, only 1 out of 22 patients with less than 20 organisms/ml of blood would have yielded a *positive* culture. Also, only 22 of 39 patients with more than 20 but less than 100 organisms/ml of blood would have been found positive. In short, only 23 of 61 patients with less than 100 organisms/ml of blood would have been considered positive by the laboratory even when three separate blood cultures were collected. Contrasting these figures with the 121 positive cultures obtained from the 121 patients, when *both* Liquoid and sucrose were added to the base medium, it seems that these two additives have an important role in the recovery of organisms in a blood culture system. What do these two additives do to allow such a dramatic increase in the incidence of positive recoveries?

If we approach the question of blood cultures with the supposition that once the blood is added to the blood culture system everything stops except the eventual multiplication of the organisms present, then there should be no difference in the incidence of recovery from any type of blood culture system utilized. As indicated by the results of this study and those of a previous study (2), this is not the case at all. In the circulating blood of the human host any bacterial cell can be challenged by phagocytes, non-specific antibody, specific antibody and/or antimicrobical agents. The question which must be answered is how much damage to a given bacterial cell can any or all of these agents do and do they continue to act once in the blood culture system? The continued action of many of the antimicrobial agents on organisms in the blood culture system has been demonstrated by many investigators. The use of such additives as penicillinase, magnesium sulfate and Liquoid (4, 5) effectively inactivate many of the antimicrobial agents. However, the simple dilution of the blood 1:10 with the base medium is usualy thought to be sufficient to render the concentration of any antimicrobial agent carried over into the blood culture system too low to effect any bacteria.

Wright (1) as well as other investigators (6, 7) have demonstrated the ability of phagocytes to continue their phagocytic activity in the blood culture system for up to 24 hours. Since the number of organisms/ml of circulating blood is usually much less than the number of phagocytes, the continued action of the phagocytes in the blood culture system could represent a major threat to the organisms. This is especially true when the bacteria are in their lag phase of growth. The presence of large numbers of active phagocytes and relatively few bacteria can lead to a

TABLE 5-IV

NUMBER OF PATIENTS POSITIVE, BY ORGANISM

Organism	Patients
Streptococcus, viridans group	41
Streptococcus pneumoniae	34
β hemolytic streptococci	12
Bacteroides	11
Streptococcus, anaerobic	9
Neisseria meningitidis	5
Haemophilus	4
Staphylococcus aureus	3
Pasteurella	2

TABLE 5-V

NUMBER OF RECOVERIES OF VARIOUS ORGANISMS BASED
ON QUANTITATIVE RESULTS*

Organism	Quantitative Group			Total
	Group I	Group II	Group III	Positive
Streptococcus, viridans group	—	12	29	41
Streptococcus pneumoniae	—	6	28	34
Streptococci, β hemolytic	2**	10	—	12
Bacteroides	3	8	—	11
Streptococci, anaerobic	7	2	—	9
Neisseria meningitidis	4	1	—	5
Haemophilus	4	—	—	4
Staphylococcus aureus[d]	—	—	3	3
Pasteurella-like organisms	2	—	—	2

---
*: Total of 121 patients.
**: Number of patients.
a: < 20 organisms/ml blood.
b: 20-99 organisms/ml blood.
c: > 100 organisms.
d: mannitol and coagulase positive.

TABLE 5-VI

NUMBER OF RECOVERIES OF VARIOUS ORGANISMS
FROM THREE TEST MEDIA

Organism	Media			Total
	Flask I[a]	Flask II[b]	Flask III[c]	Positive
Streptococcus, viridans group	37	41	41	41
Streptococcus pneumoniae	24	34	34	34
Streptococci, β hemolytic	10	12	12	12
Bacteroides	—	6	11	11
Streptococci, anaerobic	—	6	9	9
Neisseria meningitidis	—	2	5	5
Haemophilus	—	1	4	4
Staphylococcus aureus[d]	3	3	3	3
Pasteurella-like organisms	—	1	2	2

---
a: Basal medium.
b: Base medium + sodium polyanethol sulfonate.
c: Base medium + sodium polyanethol sulfonate + sucrose, 30%.
d: Mannitol and coagulase positive.

positive culture becoming negative (1). Since Liquoid disrupts the phagocytes and thus eliminates the problem of continued phagocytosis, it must be given serious consideration in any blood culture system.

von Haebler (7) and others (8, 9, 10, 11, 12, 13, 14, 15, 16, 17, 18) have shown the continued bactericidal action of complement on organisms in the blood culture system. These same investigators have also noted the continued effect of specific

TABLE 5-VII

COMPARISON OF QUANTITATIVE RECOVERIES IN THREE MEDIA

	Number of Patients in Which Either Flask I[a] or II[b] Showed at Least 30% Fewer Organisms than Flask III	Flask III[c]
Streptococcus, viridans group	12 (All > 20 but < 100)	12 (All > 100)
Streptococcus pneumoniae	6 (All > 20 but < 100)	4 (All > 100)
Streptococci, β hemolytic	12 (2 < 20)	8 (2 > 50)
	(10 > 20 but < 100)	(6 > 100)
Bacteroides	11 (3 < 20)	2 (> 100)
	(8 > 20 but < 100)	
Streptococci, anaerobic	9 (7 < 20)	7 (> 100)
	(2 > 20 but < 100)	

------

a: Base medium.
b: Base medium + sodium polyanethol sulfonate, 0.05%.
c: Base medium + sodium polyanethol sulfonate, 0.05% + sucrose, 30%.

antibody on organisms in various blood culture system. Like the activity of phagocytes, these two factors could have a major influence on the number of bacteria which survive in a blood culture system. The above quoted investigators have also found that Liquoid is able to inactivate both complement and specific antibody in blood culture systems. In addition to the above mentioned attributes of Liquoid, it is also an excellent anticoagulant. As shown by Ellner (19), as many as 90 percent of the organisms present in a blood culture system can be entrapped in a forming clot and, once entrapped, they either may die or produce micro-colonies which will be overlooked. This can be a serious problem in those laboratories that still use visible evidence of growth in the blood culture flask as the sole criterion for subculture. Hoare (20) and others (19, 21) reported that Liquoid was toxic to many bacterial species. The concentration of Liquoid used by these investigators however, was 10 times the concentration recommended by the manufacturer and used by this and other (7, 16, 22, 23, 24, 25, 26, 27, 28, 29, 30, 31 and 32) investigators. According to these latter investigators, Liquoid is non-toxic to all bacteria, when used in a final concentration of 0.05 percent (with a few possible exceptions, such as some anaerobic streptococci).

The addition of Liquoid to a blood culture system eliminates clot formation, phagocytosis and the bactericidal action of complement. If these were the only factors influencing the incidence of recovery of organisms from a blood culture system, then the use of Liquoid should allow the laboratory to have reached the ultimate in the recovery of organisms. The results of this study and of a previous study (3) indicate that the addition of Liquoid is not the final answer, since there were a greater number of positive recoveries in the test flasks containing both Liquoid and sucrose. It would appear that the addition of sucrose to a base medium containing Liquoid produces a better environment for the bacteria than the addition of Liquoid alone. There are two possible reasons for this: (1) When sucrose and Liquoid are both added to a good quality base broth, they may act together as a growth stimulator for the bacteria. (2) Each additive may have a separate effect on the environment and the combination of the separate effects produces a secure environment for the bacterial cell.

If both additives act together as a growth stimulant, then it should be possible to demonstrate this using artifically inoculated blood cultures in which the number of organisms used as the inoculum is quantitated. For this purpose, 40 sets of flasks identical to the sets used in the study were employed. They were divided into 4 groups of 10 sets each. Each group was inoculated with a different organism (obtained from positive clinical blood cultures). The first group was inoculated with a two hour broth culture of streptococci of the viridans group in such a manner as to produce a final concentration of 50 organisms/ ml of blood culture at the time of inoculation. The second group of flasks received *Streptococcus pneumoniae,* the third group beta hemolytic streptococci and the fourth group anaerobic organisms. All flasks were also inoculated with blood obtained from healthy donors. The pour plates were prepared from each flask after four hours of incubation. There were no significant differences in the number of organisms recovered from any of the test flasks regardless of the organism used. This would appear to indicate that the Liquoid/sucrose mixture did not act as a growth stimulant, for if it had, the number of organisms recovered from the Liquoid/sucrose flask would have been greater than the number recovered from the other two flasks. This small study raises some important questions, namely, why did growth occur equally well in the plain broth and the additive broths in the artificially inoculated cultures, but not in the clinical cultures? Since the organisms used as the inoculum were obtained from clinical blood cultures where they demonstrated different rates of growth in the various media, why did they grow equally well in the artificially inoculated blood cultures? Does phagocytosis occur in such an artifically inoculated blood culture system, does complement act and does specific antibody act in the same manner as shown in a clinical blood culture? This question must be answered if we are to consider as valid the results published from artifically inoculated blood culture systems. Such a study is now under way in this laboratory.

Since it appears that sucrose does not act as a growth stimulant, it must therefore have some effect on the environment in which the bacterial cell is placed. The concept of investigators working with so-called *transitional* forms or L-forms of bacteria deals with the effect of changes in osmotic pressure on bacteria that have sustained cell wall damage, may be applicable here. One factor which is often overlooked in the development of a blood culture system is the physical condition of the bacterial cells as they are placed into the system. Bacteria, like other living cells, undergo various stages of physical and biochemical deterioration in the process of dying. The rate and mode of death, to a great extent, are determined by the environment in which the cell finds itself. As already discussed, in the blood of the human host, the bacterial cell is constantly confronted by several adverse factors, such as phagocytes, complement, specific antibody and possibly specific antimicrobial agents.

Any of these factors may be capable of destroying or damaging a given bacterial cell rapidly. Since it has been shown that some of the antimicrobial agents, as well as complement and some specific antibodies, act either directly or indirectly on the bacterial cell wall, it would be safe to assume that in the circulating blood of a patient with bacteremia there will be a certain percentage of the bacterial cells in various stages of cell wall deterioration. Placing such a blood specimen into an artificial environment such as a blood culture system can place an additional stress on bacteria with cell wall defects, in the form of a sharp change in osmotic pressure. Those bacterial cells with sufficient cell wall damage will be destroyed in such a situation, as has been shown by those investigators working with either cell-wall deficient bacteria or bacteria with extreme cell wall destruction. Use of an osmotic stabilizer may prevent the destruction of these severely damaged cells. If one assumes that the cell-wall defective bacterial cell represents an advanced stage in the death process of this cell and that it has an absolute requirement for an osmotic stabilizer such as sucrose, then a bacterial cell with less cell-wall damage has a better chance of surviving in an osmotically controlled medium. This does not mean that a cell with slight or even moderate cell-wall damage requires an osmotically controlled medium, but merely, that it has a better chance of surviving and recovering in such a medium. This can become a very important consideration in those patients demonstrating very few organisms in their circulating blood.

In a previous study (3) this investigator demonstrated that the use of a sucrose broth medium did not produce an increase in the incidence of positive recoveries when compared to a plain broth medium. This was probably due to the continued action of phagocytes and/or complement since no Liquoid was included. When Liquoid was included, however, these same blood cultures demonstrated a significant increase in the incidence of recovery of organisms. It appears from the results of these studies that any blood culture system which does not include both an osmotic stabilizer such as sucrose, and an anticoagulant with additional properties such as Liquoid, will only allow the laboratory to recover organisms from those patients having a rather large number of intact bacteria/ml of blood. If this is true, then it should not only be possible for the laboratory to recover more positive cultures from a system employing both additives, but it should also be possible to obtain a higher yield of organisms from any given positive culture. In our previous study (3) twenty patients had positive blood cultures in the flask containing both additives and negative culture results in the test flasks lacking one or both additives. In the present study, fifteen patients had positive cultures only in the flasks containing both additives. In addition, the quantitative pour plates prepared from the blood culture flasks indicated that 33 patients had at least 30 percent more organisms present in the flask containing both additives, than in either of the other two test flasks. Table 5-VII indicates the organisms involved and the number of organisms recovered from each test flask. Since the organisms were in their lag phase of growth when the pour plates were prepared and the flasks were all inoculated with aliquots from the same blood sample, it can only be assumed that the higher number of organisms present in the test flasks containing both additives, was due to the adidtives acting in such a manner as to protect these cells with slight or moderate cell wall damage and that such cells were destroyed in the other two test flasks.

CONCLUSIONS

The results of this study indicate that there are two important factors which must be considered in the development of a blood culture system. The first is a method for elimination of the continued action of phagocytes, complement, and antimicrobial agents, and prevention of clot formation. Liquoid protects both the intact and cell-wall damaged cell from the above mentioned factors. The second factor is the physical condition of the bacterial cells at the time they are introduced into the blood culture system. It appears that in the circulating blood of a patient with a bacteremia there may be present a certain percentage of bacterial cells in various stages of cell-wall deterioration. The addition of an osmotic stabilizer such as sucrose, will protect these cell-wall damaged bacteria from abrupt changes in osmotic pressure, thus allowing the laboratory to recover a larger number of organisms. Wright (1) concluded that the prolongation of the lag phase in many of his cultures was due to unknown peculiarities of the organisms and was erratic. It is possible that some of his patients had a larger percentage of cell-wall damaged bacteria than intact bacteria in their blood and therefore, either the time needed to repair themselves was extended before such cells could go into the logarithmic growth phase, or the cell-wall defective forms were destroyed, leaving very few intact cells which required extended periods of time before demonstrating visible evidence of growth.

REFERENCES

1. Wright, H. D.: The bacteriology of subacute infective endocarditis. *J Pathol Bacteriol, 25*:541, 1925.
2. Rosner, R.: Effect of various anticoagulants and no anticoagulant on ability to recover bacteria directly from parallel clinical blood specimens. *Am J Clin Path, 49*:216, 1968.
3. Rosner, R.: Comparison of a blood culture system containing Liquoid and sucrose with systems containing either reagent alone. *Appl Microbiol, 19*:281, 1970.
4. Traub, W. H.: Antagonism of Polymyxin B and Kanamycin Sulfate by Liquoid (Sodium Polyanetholsulfonate) *in vitro. Experientia, 25*:206, 1969.
5. Traub, W. H., and Lowrance, B. L.: Media-dependent antagonism of gentamicin sulfate by Liquoid (Solium Polyanetholsulfonate). *Experientia, 25*:1134, 1969.
6. Van der Hoeden, J.: The influence of 'Liquoid-Roche' on the phagocytosis of brucella organisms in the blood of man and various animals. *Acta Brev Neerl, 12*:18, 1942.
7. von Haebler, T., and Miles, A. A.: The action of sodium polyanethol sulphonate ('Liquoid') on blood cultures. *J Pathol Bacteriol, 46*:245, 1938.
8. Battistini, G.: Sui rapporti tra coagulazione del sanque e complemento. *Fisiol Med, 3*:245, 1932.
9. Klein, P.: The concept of complement poisons in the anticoagulant class. *Klin Wochschr, 34*:333-334, 1956.
10. Kradolfer, F.: Einfluss von Antikoagulanten auf Zellkernproteine. *Experientia, 8*:186, 1952.
11. Lambert, H. P., and Richley, J.: The action of mucin in promoting infections: The anticomplementary effect of mucin extracts and certain other substances. *Brit J Exptl Pathol, 33*:327, 1952.
12. Lowrance, B. L., and Traub, W. H.: Inactivation of the bacteriocidal activity of human serum by Liquoid. *Appl Microbiol, 17*:839, 1969.
13. Naff, G. B., and Ratnoff, O. D.: The activation of the C'Is fragment of the first component of complement by its C'Ir fragment. *J Lab Clin Med, 70*:873, 1967.
14. Penfold, J. B.; Goldman, J., and Fairbrother, R. W.: Blood culture and selection of media. *Lancet, 1*:65-68, 1940.
15. Pontieri, G. M., and Plascia, O. J.: The comparison of methods for

the inactivation of the third component of guinea-pig complement. *Experientia, 21*:81, 82, 1965.

16. Rudolph, W.: Culture of pathogenic bacteria in the circulating blood. *Ztschr. Immunitaetsf, 95*:8, 1939.

17. Van der Hoeden, J.: De Toepassing van het verschijnsel der phago-cytose vij de diagnostiek der brucellosen. I. Het gebruik van citraat en liquoid. *Tijdschr Diergeneesk, 67*:910, 1940.

18. Yourassowsky, E.: Cinetique de l'action des antibiotiques en milieu plasmatique. *Acta Clin Belg, 4*:1, 1967.

19. Ellner, P. O., and Stoessel, C. J.: The role of temperature and anti-coagulant on the *in vitro* survival of bacteria in blood. *J Infect Disease, 116*:238, 1966.

20. Hoare, B. D.: The suitability of 'Liquoid' for use in blood culture media, with particular reference to anaerobic streptococci. *J Pathol Bacteriol, 48*:576, 1939.

21. Garrod, P. R.: The growth of *Streptococcus viridans* in sodium poly-anethol sulfonate (Liquoid). *J Pathol Bacteriol, 91*:621, 1966.

22. Evans, G. L.; Cekoric, T., and Searcy, R. L.: Comparative effects of anticoagulants on bacterial growth in experimental blood cultures. *Am J Med Tech, 34*:103, 1968.

23. Evans, G. L.; Cekoric, T.; Searcy, R. L., and Hines, L. R.: Studies on the growth of bacteria in simulated blood cultures. *Bacteriol Proc,* 1967.

24. Evans, G. L.; Cekoric, T.; Searcy, R. L., and Hines, L.: Effects of anticoagulants on antibacterial action of blood. *Clin Res, 14*:484, 1966.

25. Finegold, S. M.; Ziment, I.; White, M. L.; Winn, W. P., and Carter, W. T.: Evaluation of polyanethol sulfonate (Liquoid) in blood cultures. *Intersci Conf Antimicrobial Agents and Chemotherapy,* 7th, Oct. 25-27, Chicago, Ill., pp.59-60, 1967.

26. Fischer, K. D.: Untersuchungen ueber die Verwendung von poly-anetholsulfosaurem Natrium (Liquoid) in der bakteriologischen Blutkulturtechnik. *Thesis,* Wuerzburg, 1967.

27. Fraser, R. S.; Rossall, R. E., and Dvorkin, J.: Bacterial endocarditis occurring after open-heart surgery. *Can Med Assoc J, 96*:1551, 1967.

28. Khairat, O.: The non-aerobes of post-extraction bacteremia. *J Dental Res, 45*:1191, 1966.

29. Massa, M., and Battistini, G.: Einfaches und erfolgreiches Verfahren zur Blutzuechtung und direkter bakterioskopischer Nachweis im Blut. *Zentr Bakteriol Parasitenk, 131*:241, 1934.

30. Silver, H., and Sonnenwirth, A. C.: A practical and efficacious method of obtaining significant post mortem blood cultures. *Am J Clin Path, 52*:433, 1969.

31. Speller, D. C. E.; Prout, B. J., and Saunders, C. F.: Subacute bacterial endocarditis caused by a micro-organism resembling *Haemophilus aphrophilus. J Pathol Bacteriol,* 95:191, 1968.
32. Wilson, T. S., and Stuart, R. D.: *Staphylococcus albus* in wound infections and in septicemia. *Can Med Assoc J,* 93:8, 1965.

CHAPTER 6

THE INFECTION HAZARD POSED BY CONTAMINATED INTRAVENOUS INFUSION FLUID

Dennis G. Maki, M.D.
Frank S. Rhame, M.D.
Donald A. Goldmann, M.D.
Gerald L. Mandell, M.D.

INTRODUCTION

Fluid replacement and the administration of drugs by the intravenous (IV) route has been routinely employed since the 1930's. The plastic cannula was introduced in 1945 (1) and was enthusiastically received, particularly as a means of facilitating prolonged cannulization at one site (2-5).

Individual case reports of infectious complications of infusion therapy soon appeared, citing both the cannula (6) and the infusion fluid (7, 8) as the immediate cause. Nevertheless, during the early and middle 1950's, the main concern with the deleterious effects of infusion therapy was directed at physicochemical phlebitis in the cannulated vein (9-13). In fact, the 1962 edition of the American Hospital Association's monograph *Control of Infections in Hospitals* did not even mention infusion therapy as a potential source of infection (14).

In 1957, Moncrief reported (15) four cases of septic thrombophlebitis with fatal septicemia due to plastic femoral catheters and demonstrated an association between the incidence of complications and the duration of continuous cannula implacement. This report was followed by a series of case reports of infusion-associated septic phlebitis. The first attempts at estimating the magnitude of these problems came in two large series

(16, 17) of cases of staphylococcal septicemia, in which it was noted that at least half of the cases were traceable to local infection at a site of venous cannulation.

Aggressive pursuit of infectious complications of IV therapy ensued primarily along four lines: (1) uncontrolled, prospective and retrospective studies of infusion devices, studying irritative and purulent phlebitis, septicemia, and catheter tip contamination, and a few controlled trials of the influence of topical antibiotics on these variables, (2) nosocomial outbreaks associated with IV therapy, (3) case reports of IV-associated infections caused by unusual pathogens, and (4) deep vein septic phlebitis, usually in burn patients. All of these studies were directed toward the cannula, generally without consideration of fluid contamination. A national symposium (18) on "Safety of Large Volume Parenteral Solutions" in 1966 dealt almost entirely with toxicologic properties and particle content.

Contamination of Intravenous Infusion Fluid*

In 1953, two cases of septicemia due to *coliforms* were reported by Michaels and Reubner (19). In both cases the infecting organism was present in *heavy* concentration in the in-use infusion system. No mechanism of contamination was documented. This work was not referenced in the American literature until 1969, when Wilmore and Dudrick (20) reported on the use of an in-line membrane filter in the infusion systems of patients receiving long-term intravenous therapy. Of 250 membrane filters, of pore size .22 micron and .45 micron, most of them in place 3 days, seven (2.8%) yielded positive bacterial cultures from the upstream surface of the membrane. There was no associated illness. The organisms were not identified or quantitated. Nor was it specified whether the patients were receiving total parenteral nutrition. Robertson (21) reported two cases of visible contamination of in-use glucose saline infusion fluid with fungi, one with *Trichoderma sp.*, the other with *Penicillium sp.* Both contaminated bottles had cracks. Fungemia was demonstrable only in the first patient; despite the lack of

---

* Excluding blood products.

symptoms attributable to fungemia both patients were treated with amphoteracin B.

In 1970, Sack (22) reported on five cases of serious but non-fatal septicemia arising post-operatively in 1968. While anesthetized each of the patients received succinyl choline from an IV bottle later shown to be contaminated with *Klebsiella pneumoniae* and *Aerobacter cloacae*. There was no clouding of the solution in the bottle. The succinyl choline had been added to the bottle of dextrose 5% in Ringer's lactate on the morning it was used. The mechanism of contamination was not determined. Sack also described a similar, later case of *Klebsiella-Aerobacter* septicemia starting 1 hour after surgery. Culture of the IV solution yielded the same organisms, and the IV bottle was shown to have a crack at its base. In the same year, the first articles (23, 24) describing the infection hazard associated with total parenteral nutrition were published. Most observers had not felt that contaminated solution played a role in this complication, in part because of the frequent use of in-line membrane filters.

The first reports of systematic microbiologic examinations of in-use IV systems were published in 1971. These studies readily demonstrated that, despite the presumed sterility of these products as they arrive at the hospital, they are not necessarily sterile. The first of these studies, by Duma, Warner, and Dalton (25), was prompted by three cases of non-fatal septicemia occurring, without apparent cause, in patients receiving Abbott infusion fluids. In each case, the same species of organism as caused the septicemia was isolated from the in-use volume control set. The responsible organisms were *Escherichia sp.* in two cases and *Klebsiella sp.* in the third case. A fourth case, due to Enterobacter, was thought to have been caused in the same manner. On July 8 and 9, 1970, the group cultured 68 in-use sets. Twenty-four (35%) were contaminated with 34 organisms; 20 (59%) were gram-negative. Three of these were Enterobacter. The survey results probably were not influenced by the national outbreak of septicemia associated with Abbott IV fluids (see below), as less than 1 percent of the Abbott bottles in use at the time used the new elastomer lined cap. There was a strong correlation between the rate of contamination and the length of time the infusion system had been in use. Two additional cases, found in the survey, were described.

The second such study (26), conducted from November 1969 through December 1970, examined 1.5-3.0 ml samples from 85 in-use hyperalimentation solutions and 236 other in-use intravenous solutions. Of the former, 38 percent were contaminated, mostly with Candida (23/32), and of the latter, 9 (3.8%) were contaminated, mostly with gram-negative bacteria (7/9). No quantitation of contamination levels per bottle or clinical data were supplied. Fifty-five other bottles of hyperalimentation solution were prepared as usual, stored under various circumstances and microbiologically sampled. All were sterile, implying that contamination was occurring on the ward rather than at the time of compounding.

We at the Center for Disease Control became involved in this area in the course of characterizing a nationwide outbreak of septicemia due to intrinsic contamination of intravenous solutions made by one manufacturer (27-32). In the summer of 1970, Abbott Laboratories began the gradual switchover to a new elastomer liner in the screw cap used in their IV bottle closures. That fall and winter, many hospitals using Abbott IV fluids began to note new cases of septicemia due to *E. agglomerans* (33) (formerly called *Erwinia herbicola-lathyri*) and an increase in nosocomial septicemia due to *E. cloacae*. All of the involved patients were receiving intravenous fluids at the time of illness. CDC investigations in 25 of these hospitals demonstrated 412 cases meeting epidemiologic criteria for inclusion in the epidemic tabulations (30). In the study hospitals where in-use fluid being administered to a patient with septicemia was examined microbiologically, contamination of the in-use system was documented. The outbreak was abruptly terminated by an FDA recall of Abbott infusion products on March 22, 1971.

Studies at CDC demonstrated bacterial contamination of the outer surface of the liners from unopened Abbott bottles ranging up to 52 percent of certain lots (27). Although a variety of organisms was isolated, about 5 percent were the epidemic strains *E. cloacae* and *E. agglomerans*. Fluid from 13 of 1,825

(0.7%) unopened bottles was positive for the epidemic strains exclusively (29, 30). Much higher rates of fluid positivity (28, 31) were found when bottles were manipulated as they frequently are under hospital conditions (e.g. caps were removed and replaced and the bottles were shaken and allowed to stand at room temperature). Organisms of the Klebsiella-Enterobacter group were demonstrated to be capable of multiplying to levels of 10^6 per ml within 24 hours at room temperature in solutions containing commercial dextrose (27, 32).

Two additional studies performed in the course of investigating this outbreak are relevant to the present discussion. In cooperation with Jonas A. Shulman, M.D. in a large municipal hospital, 94 in-use infusion systems manufactured by Baxter Laboratories were cultured by membrane filtration. Administration sets or fluid of approximately 10 percent of the systems contained microorganisms in low numbers. As previously noted by Duma (25), fluid from administration sets in use longer than 48 hours was significantly more frequently contaminated than from sets in use less than 48 hours.

A second study, conducted in February 1970, at the University of Virginia Hospital prospectively compared the Abbott system with the screwcap closure (since recalled) and the Cutter system, which has a rubber bung entered by a piercing pin (now also used by Abbott). Each patient requiring infusion therapy was randomly assigned to one brand for the duration of his therapy. All systems were cultured daily by removing the entire infusion system, except for the cannula, and subjecting the fluid in each component, separately, to membrane filtration. During the study period, Abbott systems showed a rate of overall in-use contamination (20.0%) nearly threefold greater than Cutter (6.8%), and *E. cloacae, E. agglomerans* or indol-positive *Klebsiella* were isolated from 8 Abbott systems and only one Cutter. Most impressive, no patients became clinically infected, although in seven instances contamination was *heavy* (confluent growth on millipore filter membrane). The lack of symptoms, despite IV receiving fluids with more than 300 organisms per 100 ml, was attributed to a daily change of each patient's administration set.

A fundamental concept in analyzing the hazard of contaminated IV fluid was developed during the investigation of the outbreak. The organisms involved were organisms of low pathogenicity which, in the low numbers usually present after initial extrinsic contamination, would normally not be dangerous, even when injected intravenously. To achieve clinical significance, these organisms must be able to multiply in the particular solution. On the basis of the limited data now available, there appears to be a remarkable degree of specificity associated with this capability. For dextrose 5% in water, only members of the tribe Klebsiellae, such as *Enterobacter cloacae, E. agglomerans* and *Klebsiella pneumoniae,* are able to multiply. Over 50 randomly selected clinical isolates from this tribe, washed twice to remove residual organic nitrogen, inoculated into dextrose 5% in water and incubated at 25°C, attained a mean normalized 24 hour concentration of over 10^5 organisms per ml. There was no turbidity or other visual evidence of microbial growth. In contrast, 51 randomly selected strains of *Staphylococcus, Pseudomonas, Proteus, E. coli,* and *Herellea,* one *Herellea* strain, died or did not grow. The inability to grow is probably due to the acid pH of commercial dextrose in water and the absence of an organic nitrogen source. The only organisms capable of growing in hyperalimentation fluid, which is acid and hypertonic, are Candida (26, 34) and Torulopsis, although some bacteria may be able to grow slowly. A complete list of the organisms capable of growing in each solution type might help the clinician faced with choosing an antibiotic for a patient with septicemia suspected of being caused by fluid.

Sources of Extrinsic Contamination

Contamination may occur at any of the many connections in the infusion apparatus (Figure 6-1). Probably the most important source of in-use contamination is by direct contact of system components with the hands of personnel and unsterile environmental surfaces. Confirmation of the importance of these sources is provided by the observation that more complex systems tend to be contaminated more frequently (25), and contamination increases with duration of use (25). Over 20 percent of

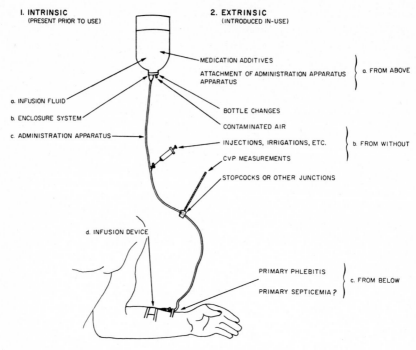

Figure 6-1. Potential mechanisms for bacterial contamination of IV infusion fluids.

hospital personnel carry antibiotic-resistant coliforms on their hands (35), and randomly sampled creams frequently used after handwashing are often heavily contaminated by Candida (36) and Klebsiella-Enterobacter organisms (37).

When used properly, neither the Viaflex bag, which needs no air to displace the solution, nor the Cutter or Abbott systems admit unfiltered air into the IV bottle. Provided air filters are not wetted, they should adequately remove airborne microbial particles from entering air. The Travenol and McGaw 1-liter bottles allow an in-rush of about 150 ml of unfiltered air at the time of removal of the thin rubber wafer. The liter of air entering thereafter, although unfiltered, is probably much less hazardous because it enters a down pointing, 20 cm inlet tube. To reach the inside of the bottle it would have to settle at a rate slower than air moving up the tube but fast enough to reach the fluid after entrance. It is possible to estimate the potential hazard of the initial 150 ml of unfiltered air. Hospital air contains about 25 colony forming units (CFU) per cubic foot (38) (although the air in the immediate vicinity of the hand removing the wafer may be more heavily contaminated); this is about 1 CFU per liter or .15 CFU per 150 ml. The initial in-rush of air might be expected to contribute organisms to about 15 percent of the bottles. About 25 percent of the organisms in hospital air are gram-negative bacteria or yeasts (39), the organism of concern as IV fluid contaminants. One study (40) did find a higher rate of contamination in *open* than in *closed* systems.

The contribution of air has been studied by Perceval (41), who analyzed contamination levels in bottles using a closure system with a removable latex wafer (such as Travenol and McGaw now use). His experiments were performed in a room where the air had been artificially contaminated with an aerosolized solution of *Staphylococcus albus* at a level "fairly high, but not unattainable on wards." In this circumstance, many bacteria entered the bottle with the in-rush of air at the time the diaphragm was removed, but none were present if the vacuum was first broken by a needle with an airway filter. The rate of this occurrence in normal air was not established. The demonstration of in-use contamination in systems using air filters (34, 39) indicates that air is not the only source of contamination.

In an analysis of particulate matter in infusion fluid, Garvan and Gunner (42), reporting from Australia, found fungal elements in 40 percent of the units sampled. They documented a "high incidence of fungal contamination of natural raw rubber" and felt that fungi reached the fluid from *blisters* on the rubber bung and by *coring* or trauma of the bung during introduction of the pin of the administration set. Since their reports, all U.S. manufacturers have begun using coated (usually lacquered) bungs, thus reducing this source of contamination.

Hairline cracks have been implicated in several of the cited clinical cases (21, 22), but this is clearly not responsible for the bulk of in-use contamination.

Retrograde contamination from organisms in the blood remains an intriguing theoretical possibility. After insertion, catheters are rapidly coated with coagulation products (43) that can serve to support microbial growth. Catheter tips, even after aseptic removal (43, 44), frequently harbor organisms. Furthermore, microorganisms can move vertically more than 5 feet in Foley catheter tubing against gravity and a continuous flow of fluid (46). Contamination of bottles from fluid lines could readily be accomplished during bottle change by squeezing drip chambers. However, when in-line filters were cultured, microorganisms were only seen on the upstream side of the filters (20, 24).

Control of Fluid Contamination

The nationwide epidemic of nosocomial septicemia caused by intrinsically contaminated Abbott intravenous products was a one-time event. The prevention of intrinsic contamination (Fig. 6-1) is a problem for the manufacturers and regulatory agencies rather problem for the manufacturers and regulatory agencies rather than the clinician. The USP regulations in effect at the time of the outbreak required microbiological sampling of 10 ml of 10 bottles of a given lot (such lots usually contain between 5,000 and 30,000 bottles). If any growth was noted, an additional 20 units were sampled; the lot was rejected if contamination was again found. Identification of contaminants is not required. This sampling procedure would pass 98 percent of lots in which one bottle out of 100 was contaminated. Although current USP standards require an initial examination of 20 units in each lot, 96 percent of such lots will still pass inspection. In fact, it is impractical to sample enough units to ensure the sterility of any given lot. For example, approximately 10 percent of a 3,000 unit lot would have to be sampled to establish with 95 percent confidence that the contamination level is less than one per hundred. However, the value of sterility testing can be increased by identifying contaminants, at least to the genus level. Such a procedure, over a period of time, would give meaningful information about manufacturing processes. For example, isolation of *E. agglomerans, E. cloacae,* and other pathogens from even a few bottles of unused intravenous fluid should probably prompt an early review of manufacturing technique. When a change in infusion system is introduced, manufacturers must test it in as close to the in-use situation as possible. Provided the infusion system design is adequate, the sterility of a given lot of intravenous fluids can be practically assured only by monitoring the sterilization process (e.g. recording thermocouples to document acceptable autoclaving temperatures).

Nationwide epidemics of nosocomial infection caused by contaminated products may, in the future, be recognized early by the National Nosocomial Infections Study (NNIS), a program to analyze the output from the nosocomial infection surveillance programs of selected hospitals (47).

Central IV additive services are becoming increasingly prevalent in the nation's hospitals and have been advocated as a means of reducing contamination. Contamination due to airborne microorganisms should be reduced by mixing IV fluids in a laminar air flow hood (48). Adherence to strict asepsis is probably greater in a pharmacy than on the hectic ward where nurses have many different tasks.

However, although central IV additive services offer undisputed advantages, such as reduction of dosage and medication errors, prevention of drug incompatibility, and increased adherence to rational therapeusis (49), controlled studies have not yet been performed to demonstrate the usefulness of such services in reducing intravenous fluid contamination and the resulting clinical disease. One study (50) showed that preparation of hyperalimentation fluid in a pharmacy's laminar flow hood did not completely eliminate contamination during preparation; 2.5 percent of samples tested were contaminated even before they left the laminar flow hood. Another study (26) indicates that careful technique in the pharmacy cannot be expected to significantly reduce the incidence of contamination, since most contamination occurs after the fluid leaves the pharmacy. Also, laminar air flow hoods require careful maintenance (50). Furthermore, if central IV additive services bring an increase in the time between first opening bottles and administration to the patient, there might be an overall increase in hazard even though fewer bottles become contaminated. Storing bottles at 4°C (36) may enable an extension of the 24-hour rule (see below), but additional problems arise when the bottles return to room temperature; cold bottles *sweat* allowing moisture to accumulate that could contaminate the area of insertion of piercing pins. Expanding bottle contents may, under some circumstances, force fluid out air filters (reducing their effectiveness) or air inlets.

Efforts of manufacturers and regulatory agencies to produce a sterile product will be confounded at the bedside unless scrupulous antiseptic technique is employed when preparing and administering intravenous fluids. Hands should be thoroughly washed before preparing solutions and manipulating infusion apparatus. Volume control devices, *piggy-backs*, monometers, stopcocks, and other apparatus should be employed only when necessary and should be removed as soon as clinically warranted. Hands should be washed before all patient contact and the utmost care should be taken to maintain asepsis during all manipulations of IV apparatus. Some have advocated the application of an antimicrobial agent at the junctions of the various components of the infusion apparatus. Without a demonstrated mechanism of contamination providing a theoretical rationale or a controlled prospective trial, the authors cannot recommend this precaution.

In-line microbial filters theoretically offer an excellent solution to the problem; they are now employed in most of the nation's total parenteral nutrition programs. In the reported instances of microbial growth on the upstream surface of these filters no clinical septicemia occurred (20, 24). Nor should the value of removing particulate matter be overlooked (51). But it has been pointed out that some aberrant bacterial forms may be able to pass even the .22 micron pore size filters (52). Final filters are untested, as yet, in a controlled trial, and they pose the drawbacks of expense, inconvenience, diminution of flow rates, and the addition of yet another manipulation to the system.

A corollary of the principle that to become clinically significant, contaminants must be capable of multiplying in the particular contaminated solution is that the solution must be contaminated long enough for such proliferation to occur. In dextrose solutions members of the tribe Klebsielleae, require about 24 hours at room temperature to reach levels of 10^5 per ml after inoculation at about 1 per ml (32). Thus, no IV bottle should be kept in place more than 24 hours. Keep-open IV's should not use bottles larger than 250 ml to ensure adherence to this point. Furthermore, the entire infusion apparatus, down to the cannula, should be changed at the time of a bottle change every 24 hours. At the time of routine cannula change, an entirely new bottle and administration apparatus should be used.

Most phlebitis associated with intravenous cannulation is due to physicochemical irritation (53). In solutions of dextrose, a substantial cause of this irritation arises from the acid pH (54) needed to prevent caramelization during autoclaving. These observations are relevant to infection control in two ways. Neutralizing the solution after autoclaving requires an additional additive which increases the potential for contamination, and the spectrum of organisms capable of multiplying in the solution would probably be extended, particularly to the Pseudomonads.

A discussion of other recommendations (55) dealing with prevention of infusion-therapy-associated infection, directed at the skin-cannula area, is not within the scope of this paper. It is probable that all such recommendations plus those outlined here will be better adhered to by an IV team, whose special duty it is to insert and maintain infusion devices. Such a team is particularly important for total parenteral nutrition (56), where the infection hazard may assume alarming proportion (57).

A wider appreciation of the hazards of contaminated IV solutions should lead to inclusion of this etiology in the differential diagnosis when a patient receiving IV fluids has clinical septicemia with no apparent primary source. In such a situation, in addition to the usual measures for evaluating the patient, an entirely new infusion system should be substituted and the old system should be cultured using broth and a pour plate. It should be kept in mind that microbial growth has not been visible in infusion systems contaminated with bacteria and that almost half such patients do not have phlebitis (30).

REFERENCES

1. Meyers, L.: Intravenous catheterization. *Am J Nurs, 45*:930-931, 1945.
2. Guenther, T. A.; Grindlay, J. H., and Lundy, J. S.: New flexible capillary tubing for use in venoclysis. *Proc Staff Meet Mayo Clinic, 22*:206-207, 1947.
3. Duffy, B. J.: The clinical use of polyethylene tubing for intravenous therapy: A report on 72 cases. *Ann Surg, 130*:929-936, 1949.
4. Erwin, P.; Strickler, J. H., and Rice, C. O.: Use of polyethylene tubing in intravenous therapy for surgical patients. *AMA Arch Surg, 66*:673-678, 1953.
5. Anderson, L. H.: Venous catheterization for fluid therapy: technique and results. *J Lab Clin Med, 36*:645-649, 1950.
6. Neuhof, H., and Seley, G. P.: Acute suppurative phlebitis complicated by septicemia. *Surg, 21*:831-842, 1947.
7. Duhig, J. V., and Mead, M.: Systemic mycosis due to *Monilia albicans. Med J Aust, 1*:179-182, 1951.
8. Geiger, A. J.; Wenner, H. A., and Axilrod, H. D., *et al.*: Mycotic endocarditis and meningitis: report of a case due to *Monilia albicans. Yale J Biol Med, 18*:259-268, 1946.
9. Anderson, L. H.; Aldrich, S. L.; Halpern, B., and Dolkart, R. E.: Venous catheterization for continuous parenteral fluid therapy. *J Lab Clin Med, 38*:585-587, 1956.
10. Editorial: Thrombophlebitis after infusions. *Lancet, 2*:541, 1955.
11. Report to Medical Research Council: Thrombophlebitis following intravenous infusions: Trial of plastic and red rubber giving-sets. *Lancet, 1*:595-597, 1957.
12. Bogen, J. E.: Local complications in 167 patients with indwelling venous catheters. *Surg Gyn Obst,* 112-114, 1960.
13. Editorial: Thrombophlebitis following intravenous infusion. *Lancet, 1*:907, 1960.
14. Colbeck, J. C., ed.: Control of infections in hospitals. *Am Hosp Assoc,* Chicago, Ill., 1962.
15. Moncrief, J. A.: Femoral catheters. *Ann Surg, 147*:166-172, 1968.
16. Collins, H. S.; Helper, A. N., and Blevins, A., *et al.*: Staphylococcal bacteremia. *Ann New York Acad Sci, 05*:222-234, 1956.
17. Hassall, J. E., and Rountree, P. M.: Staphylococcal septicemia. *Lancet, 1*:213-217, 1959.
18. Food and Drug Administration: Proceedings of the National Symposium: Safety of large volume parenteral solutions, Washington, D.C., July 28-29, 1966.
19. Michaels, L., and Ruebner, B.: Growth of bacteria in intravenous infusion fluids. *Lancet, 1*:772-774, 1953.

20. Wilmore, D. W., and Dudrick, S. J.: An in-line filter for intravenous solutions. *Arch Surg, 99*:462-463, 1969.
21. Robertson, M. H.: Fungi in fluids—a hazard of intravenous therapy. *J Med Microbiol, 3*:99-102, 1970.
22. Sack, R. A.: Epidemic of gram-negative organism septicemia subsequent to elective operation. *Am J Obstet Gynec, 107*:394-399, 1970.
23. Boeckman, C. R., and Krill, C. E.: Bacterial and fungal infections complicating parenteral alimentation in infants and children. *J Ped Surg, 5*:117-126, 1970.
24. Ashcraft, K. W., and Leape, L. L.: *Candida* sepsis complicating parenteral feeding. *J Am Med Assoc, 212*:454-456, 1970.
25. Duma, R. J.; Warner, J. E., and Dalton, H. P.: Septicemia from intravenous infusions. *New Engl J Med, 257*-275, 1971.
26. Deeb, E. N., and Natsios, C. A.: Contamination of intravenous fluids by bacteria and fungi during preparation and administration. *Am J Hosp Pharm, 28*:764-767, 1971.
27. Center for Disease Control: Nosocomial bacteremias associated with intravenous fluid therapy—USA. *Morbidity & Mortality Weekly Rep, 20*: Special supplement to No. 6, 1971.
28. Center for Disease Control: Follow-up on septicemias associated with contaminated Abbott intravenous solutions—United States. *Morbidity & Mortality Weekly Rep, 20*:91-92, 1971.
29. Center for Disease Control: Follow-up on septicemia associated with contaminated intravenous fluid from Abbott Laboratories. *Morbidity & Mortality Weekly Rep, 20*:110, 1971.
30. Maki, D. G.; Rhame, F. S., and Mackel, D. C., *et al.*: Nationwide epidemic of septicemia caused by contaminated intravenous fluid: I. Epidemiologic and clinical features. Manuscript in preparation.
31. Mackel, D. C.; Maki, D. G., and Anderson, R. L., *et al.*: Nationwide epidemic of septicemia caused by contaminated intravenous fluid: II. Mechanisms of intrinsic contamination. Manuscript in preparation.
32. Maki, D. G., and Martin, W. T.: Nationwide epidemic of septicemia caused by contaminated intravenous fluid: III. Studies of microbial growth in commercial intravenous fluid. Manuscript in preparation.
33. Ewing, W. H., and Fife, M. A.: *Enterobacter agglomerans.* The *herbicola-lathyri* bacteria. Center for Disease Control, Atlanta, Georgia, 1971.
34. Brennan, M. E.; O'Connell, R. C., and Rosol, J. A., *et al.*: Growth of *Candida albicans* in nutritive solutions given parenterally. *Arch Surg, 103*:705-708, 1971.
35. Salzman, T. C.; Clark, J. J., and Klemm, L.: Hand contamination of personnel as a mechanism of cross-infection in nosocomial infections

with antibiotic-resistant *Escherichia coli* and *Klebsiella-aerobacter*. *Antimicrob Agents & Chemoth*, 97-100, 1967.

36. France, D. R.: Survival of *Candida albicans* in hand creams. *New Zealand Med J*, 67:552-554, 1968.

37. Morse, L. J., and Schonbeck, L. E.: Hand lotions—a potential nosocomial hazard. *New Engl J Med*, 278:376-378, 1968.

38. Greene, V. W.; Vesley, D., and Bond, R. G., *et al.*: Microbiological contamination of hospital air. II. Qualitative Studies. *Appl Microbial*, 10:567-571, 1962.

39. Greene, V. W.; Vesley, D., and Bond, R. G., *et al.*: Microbiologic contamination of hospital air. *Appl Microbiol* 10:561-566, 1962.

40. Miller, W. A.; Smith, G. L., and Latiolars, C. J.: A comparative evaluation of compounding costs and contamination rates of intravenous admixture systems. *Drug Intell Clin Pharmacy*, 5:51-52, 1971 as quoted in (49).

41. Perceval, A. K.: Contamination of parenteral solutions during administration. *Med J Australia*, 2:954-956, 1966.

42. Garvan, J. M., and Gunner, B. W.: The harmful effects of particles in intravenous fluids. *Med J Australia*, 2:1-6, 1964.

43. Jacobsson, B.; Bergentz, S. E., and Ljunqvist, V.: Platelet adhesion and thrombus formation on vascular catheters in dogs. *Acta Radiol Diag*, 8:221-227, 1969.

44. Corso, J. A.; Agostinelli, R., and Brandriss, M. W.: Maintenance of venous polyethylene catheters to reduce risk of infection. *J Am Med Assoc*, 210:2075-2077, 1969.

45. Fuchs, P. C.: Indwelling intravenous polyethylene catheters: factors influencing the risk of microbial colonization and sepsis. *J Am Med Assoc*, 216:1447-1450, 1971.

46. Weyrauch, H. M., and Bassett, J. B.: Ascending infection in an artificial urinary tract; an experimental study. *Stanford Med Bull*, 9:25-29, 1951.

47. Maki, D. G.; Scheckler, W. E., and Brachman, P., *et al.*: A national nosocomial infections surveillance study. Presented at the 98th Ann Meet APHA, Houston, Texas, Oct. 28, 1970.

48. Wahlstrom, L., and Oberg, S.: Efficiency of laminar air-flow clean benches as measured by physical and microbiological particle counting. *Drug Intelligence*, 1:158-163, 1967.

49. Engel, G.: Addition of drugs to intravenous fluids. *Med J Australia*, 2:962-966, 1971.

50. Hak, L. J.; Long, J. L., and Ruberg, R. L., *et al.*: Contamination incidence in IV solutions with additives. Presented at the Annual Meeting of the American Society of Hospital Pharmacists, March 31, 1971.

51. Davis, N. M., and Turco, S.: A study of particulate matter in IV infusion fluids—phase 2. *Am J Hosp Pharm, 28*:620-623, 1971.

52. Duma, R. J.; Warner, J. F., and Dalton, H. P.: Letter to the editor. *New Eng J Med, 284*:1038, 1971.

53. Thomas, E. T.; Evers, W., and Racz, G. B.: Postinfusion phlebitis. *Anaesthes Analges, 49*:150-159, 1970.

54. Fonkalsrud, E. W.: Neutralization of IV fluids. *New Engl J Med, 280*:1480, 1969.

55. Hospital Infections Section: Recommendations for the insertion and maintenance of plastic intravenous catheters. CDC Publication, Atlanta, Georgia, Jan. 1972.

56. Goldmann, D. A., and Maki, D. G.: A rational approach to the problem of sepsis in hyperalimentation therapy. Symposium on Total Parenteral Nutrition, Nashville, Tennessee, Am Med Assoc, Jan. 18, 1972.

57. Curry, C. R., and Quie, P. G.: Fungal septicemia in patients receiving parenteral hyperalimentation. *New Engl J Med, 285*:1221-1225, 1971.

AUTHOR INDEX

SUBJECT INDEX

A

Abscess
  hepatic, 56
Acetate, 55
Acetoin, 45
Acinetobacter (Mima-Herellea), 7, 10
Actinobacillus, 10
Actinobacillus actinomycetemcomitans,
  51, 52
Additives
  blood culture, 16, 20, 26, 27, 38, 40,
    43, 61, 62, 64-72
  infusion fluid, 82, 85, 87
Adonitol, fermentation, 55, 57
Aerobacter cloacae, 78
Aerobe, 30
  obligate, 43, 44
Aerobic bacteria, 23
Aerobic incubation, 44
Aerobic method of blood culture,
  26, 27
Aeromonas, 7, 10, 57
Agar
  blood, 21, 43, 53
  chocolate, 21, 30, 43
  Columbia Blood, 20, 63
  eosin-methylene blue, 43, 56
  Kan, 21
  MacConkey, 56
  triple sugar-iron (TSIA), 54-57
  trypticase soy, 20, 54
Agranulocytosis, 5
Air filter
  in infusion therapy, 82, 83, 84, 86
Albimi tryptose soy broth, 54
Aminoglycoside, 40, 50
Ammonium oxalate, 40
Amphotericin B., 78
Anaerobe, 23, 31, 36, 42, 44, 50-52
  isolation, 29, 32

Anaerobic bacilli, 50
Anaerobic bacteremia, 47, 51
Anaerobic bacteria, viii, 23, 43, 47, 50,
  51
Anaerobic broth culture, 42
Anaerobic incubation, 20, 63
Anaerobic method of blood culture, 9,
  20, 26, 29
Anaerobic osmotically stabilized broth,
  44
Anaerobic streptococci, 10, 38, 50, 68
Anaerobic *Streptococcus*, 7, 66, 67
Anemia, aplastic, 5
Antibiotic-resistant coliforms, 82
Antibiotic therapy, 25, 26
  and colonization rates of gram-
    negative bacilli, 5
Antibiotics, 3, 4, 11, 24, 25, 28, 29, 49,
  50, 77, 81
  resistance to, 4, 5
  susceptibility tests, 10, 11, 21, 31,
    44, 50
Antibody
  complement, 68
  non-specific, 66
  specific, 66-68, 70
Anticoagulant, 16, 26, 40, 68, 71
Antigenic patterns, of microorganisms,
  vii
Antimetabolic therapy, 5
Antimicrobial agents, 4, 10, 36, 39, 40,
  44, 66, 70, 72, 86
  susceptibility tests, 32, 42
Antimicrobial therapy, 24, 31, 50
Aplastic anemia, 5
Arabinose, fermentation, 55, 57
Arginine dihydrolase test, 55-57
Asepsis, 86
Autoclaving, 38, 85, 87

99